THE

SAFE EXERCISE

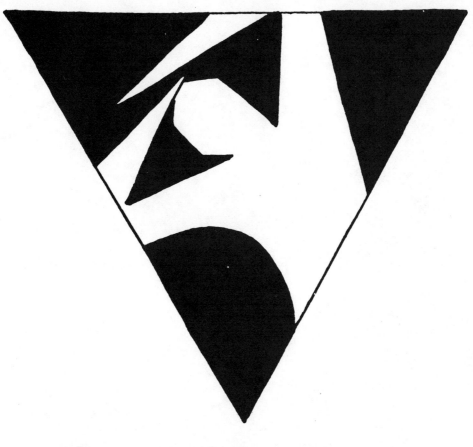

HANDBOOK

By Toni Tickel Branner

Illustrated by Nancy Ann Briggs

KENDALL/HUNT PUBLISHING COMPANY
2460 Kerper Boulevard   P.O. Box 539   Dubuque, Iowa 52004-0539

TABLE OF CONTENTS

Preface

During the past decade the public has been bombarded with information about fitness and health. Almost everyone knows that exercise is a good thing but most people have not stayed up to date on the latest research and techniques. *The Safe Exercise Handbook* was created because most of the fitness books on the market include outdated stretches and calisthenics which may contribute to low back and knee problems as well as other injuries. This book promotes the importance of a regular exercise program as a means of improving your health and quality of life. A conservative approach is utilized to assist you in designing a total workout which will accomplish your individual goals while decreasing the chance that an injury will occur.

Objectives of *The Safe Exercise Handbook*

Dispels the "no pain, no gain" and "more is better" philosophy. Exercise should not hurt.

Updates the public on current research and new concepts relating to stretching safety, proper progression, warm-up, and exercise techniques.

Promotes total wellness. Information is provided on eating for an active lifestyle, managing stress and increasing compliance to healthy behaviors.

Provides the lay public with the information necessary to carry out a safe, effective exercise program without burdening the reader with extraneous information. Most fitness books include very comprehensive material but the novice exerciser loses the "how to" information in the midst of scientific studies and complicated charts.

Target Audience

Undergraduate Fitness Classes: Test-marketed on over 1500 college students enrolled in wellness-oriented activity classes (aerobic dance, exercise and conditioning, weight training, walking, aqua-aerobics, and jogging).

Worksite Fitness and Wellness Programs: Designed as follow-up for exercise testing and health risk appraisal in supervised wellness programs. Forms for recording results of health and fitness screening as well as space for individual exercise programs and daily fitness logs are included.

Public School Resource for Physical and Health Educators: Used successfully to introduce teachers and administrators to new concepts in exercise and health. Also appropriate as a workbook for senior high students.

Patient Education for Physicians: Most physicians do not have time to thoroughly counsel each individual patient. *The Safe Exercise Handbook* is a complete, inexpensive guide to starting a conservative fitness program.

General Fitness Guide for the Lay Public: Over 80% of Americans will eventually experience low back pain. Exercise physiologists now agree that all exercisers should be put on a preventive fitness program in order to avoid chronic damage to the back and other joints. Using *The Safe Exercise Handbook* as a guide, one can achieve all the benefits of regular activity while virtually eliminating the risks.

Acknowledgements

This book was created to fill a special need. When I was hired to implement the UNC Employee Health and Fitness Center I received encouragement from faculty and staff who said they no longer hurt after exercise sessions prescribed by our staff. The time demands of individual counseling prompted the creation of this book so that each participant would have all of the information to take home with them. Credit must be extended to these dedicated employees.

Thanks also to the faculty and staff in the Department of Physical Education at UNC and my students who are so enthusiastic and interested in wellness and exercise. A special acknowledgement to Joe Miller and the faculty at the Principals' Executive Program who have allowed me to disperse this information into the public school system. The health of our educators and our children is the key to a future of wellness.

A special thank you to Nancy Briggs for the illustrations, Linda Prather for the photography, and models Aristotle Domnas, Tami Tickel and Marianne Wolf.

My husband and family deserve an award for their love and support as well as providing insight for practical evaluation of my ideas.

The basic philosophy and inspiration for *The Safe Exercise Handbook* must be credited to my mother, Rebecca Henley Brown. After teaching fitness and aerobic dance classes in our basement and at a local health spa for many years she enrolled at George Mason University to earn a B.S. in exercise science. Her business, The Exercise Studio, Inc., evolved providing safe, effective classes which were years ahead of the rest of the fitness world with regard to safety and effectiveness. Innovations in low-impact aerobic dance, instructor training and modifying for individual differences were a part of her program long before the information appeared in exercise books. As I entered the health field I was amazed at how many ineffective and contraindicated exercises were still a regular part of most fitness regimes. *The Safe Exercise Handbook* strives to reeducate this population and to show newcomers the way to lifetime, injury-free fitness.

INTRODUCTION

Most things seem to evolve or change over time, hopefully for the better. The same is true for exercise. Professionals are realizing that some of the activities, stretches, and calisthenics that we have always done may be causing chronic or acute injuries. The new philosophy in health and fitness focuses on achieving the benefits without taking on the associated risks. Although all risks cannot be eliminated, most individuals should be able to participate in a fitness routine without experiencing injury, pain or discomfort and should be able to continue this program for a lifetime. This concept is difficult for those who adhere to the "no pain, no gain" and the "more is better" philosophy.

Choosing the safest and the most effective fitness program should be the primary goal for all individuals who wish to exercise. The problems arise when people choose the older and less safe methods for the sake of tradition or simply out of habit. We now know that some of our favorite stretches and exercises are not very safe and in some cases are not very effective. Some of these may not cause discomfort initially, but over time may lead to chronic, overuse injuries.

The secret to exercising safely is moderation. Do enough to achieve the benefits without creating unnecessary stress or injury. Another key element is knowledge. The more you know about exercise principles and proper technique, the safer and more effective your workout will be. Also remember that exercising for health is much different than training for athletics. Often athletes risk injury for the sake of competition or recreation. Dancers and gymnasts place their bodies in extreme positions for competitive reasons and to create artistic images. If your goal is to be fit and healthy, there is no need to do anything which jeopardizes your body. Exercise does not have to be painful. If it hurts, leave it out!

This book promotes the importance of a regular exercise program as a means of improving your health and quality of life. A conservative approach is utilized to assist you in designing a total workout which will accomplish your individual goals while decreasing the chance that an injury will occur. A book cannot replace personal guidance from a trained exercise professional. When you have questions seek information or classes in your community or at local colleges and universities.

Medical Considerations

Before embarking on any fitness program you might want to consider a medical evaluation of your current health status. If you have been following a regular exercise routine or if you are under 35 years of age and have no significant health problems it is probably okay to begin a moderate exercise program. If, however, you have a serious medical problem, have never exercised, or are over 35 it is imperative that you consult with your physician about the possible effects of increased physical activity.

Sticking With It

This book helps each individual design an exercise plan specific to personal needs and goals. It is relatively easy to start a program, however, sticking with it long enough to gain benefits is difficult for most people. Below are some suggestions and tips to help you adhere to your healthy lifestyle changes.

Remember that exercise is not always fun or convenient. Your workout must become a habit, just like brushing your teeth. And of course, you always feel better afterward.

Make it as convenient as possible. If you have to drive twenty miles to exercise you are less likely to do it than if you can stop on the way home from work. Have an alternate plan for vacations, weekends, rainy days, or very busy times.

Utilize support systems. A friend, co-worker, or spouse can cover responsibilities for you while you exercise and you can do the same for them.

If it hurts - stop! You are unlikely to continue any activity which is painful or causes delayed muscle soreness. Seek professional advice and switch to a different activity until the injury heals.

Keep a log (see appendix) of your activity. It is motivating to look back on our accomplishments and see progress.

Don't try too much too soon. It can be overwhelming to start exercising, change your diet and quit smoking all at the same time. Write down your plan and proceed gradually. Each change will lead to a new one.

Avoid boredom, vary your workout. Try different activities, locations and exercise partners. Make exercise a family affair. Weekend hikes, cycling trips, and nature walks are wonderful.

You will have bad weeks. If you miss an exercise session, eat a banana split, or smoke a cigarette remember that it is not the end of the world. Analyze why it happened, admit that you need to do better next week and get back on target.

Reward your efforts. For example, if you stick with it for three months reward yourself with a new outfit, tennis racket, or weekend trip.

Notes

Chapter One

ACHIEVING TOTAL FITNESS

The Five Components of Fitness

Becoming totally fit requires achieving a balance between the five components of fitness. These include:

Cardiovascular Endurance
Muscular Strength
Muscular Endurance
Flexibility
Body Composition

Designing your exercise session to accommodate all of these factors will ensure maximum benefits to your health.

Cardiovascular Endurance

Exercise physiologists and other health professionals usually agree that aerobic exercise is the most important component of fitness as it relates to overall health. It is the only kind of exercise that significantly reduces the risk for heart disease and the only form of activity that burns fat as the major fuel source. The word *aerobic* means "with oxygen". Oxygen is necessary to burn the fuels which produce energy for prolonged activity. By exercising aerobically we initiate physiologic changes which increase the efficiency of the heart, lungs and circulatory system. A healthy heart has the ability to supply plenty of oxygen and nutrients to the working muscles during normal activities as well as any emergency situations which might arise.

Aerobic exercises are those that are rhythmical, continuous and involve large muscle groups. Aerobic activities such as walking, running, cycling, and aerobic dance increase the heart rate to a target level and maintain it at that level for a certain length of time. Chapter Four demonstrates how to choose an activity and how to determine the appropriate frequency, duration, and intensity of your aerobic workout.

Muscular Strength

Muscular strength is the amount of force a muscle can exert or resist for a brief period of time. Research and practical experience tell us that if we stress a muscle or muscle group more than it is normally used to, it will eventually adapt and improve its function. Therefore, certain exercises are designed to increase strength so that we may perform our everyday activities with less exertion and less chance of injury.   Likewise, if a muscle is stressed less than it is usually accustomed it will atrophy and lose strength. People with broken limbs are good examples. The limb is immobilized for a length of time and when the cast is removed, one limb is usually smaller than the other. Exercises utilizing weight training, calisthenics and stretchy bands will help to increase muscular strength.

Often individuals have sufficient strength in some muscle groups but are deficient in others. For example, we use our quadriceps (thigh muscles) everytime we walk, run, climb stairs, etc. Our hamstrings (back of the thigh) usually receive no significant exercise throughout the day. The quadriceps, therefore, are relatively stronger and pull with more force on the skeletal system. This kind of muscular imbalance is often the source of lower back pain, knee problems, and various other injuries. It can also affect your posture and movement patterns. Thus, when using strength training to improve health it is important to concentrate on the weaker areas in order to create balance. A good rule to remember is: **STRETCH THE STRONG MUSCLES AND STRENGTHEN THE WEAK ONES!**

Relatively Strong Muscles	Relatively Weak Muscles
Quadriceps/Hip Flexors	Hamstrings
Adductors (inner thigh)	Abductor (outer thigh)
Gastrocnemius (calves)	Tibialis Anterior (shins)
Pectoralis Group (chest)	Rhomboids /Upper Back
Erector Spinae	Abdominals
Biceps	Triceps

Muscular strength requirements are different for each individual. Some people need only to perform everyday tasks such as bringing in groceries while others wish to partake in vigorous sports or hard labor. Chapter Five assists you in making safe and intelligent decisions concerning your strength training.

Muscular Endurance

Muscular endurance describes the ability of muscles to sustain repeated contractions or apply sustained force against a fixed object. If having muscular strength allows you to pick up a heavy box, then having muscular endurance allows you to pick up ten boxes one after the other. Activities such as sit-ups, push-ups, raking leaves, shoveling snow and pushing a lawn mower all require prolonged muscular exertion. Chapter Five describes muscular endurance exercises which are safe and effective.

Flexibility

Flexibility is the range of motion possible around a joint. Stretching exercises are utilized to maintain or increase this range of movement, to help prevent muscle soreness, and to prevent injuries.

Since flexibility is specific to every joint, it is incorrect to refer to flexibility in a general sense (i.e. John has good flexibility). Each joint must be evaluated separately. Another common misconception is to assume that to have good flexibility a person must have an excessive amount, such as a gymnast or a dancer. Athletes and performers often place their bodies in positions which stretch muscles and connective tissue beyond the point deemed necessary for normal function. They do this for the sake of competition or aesthetics even though injuries often result.

Many people hate to stretch because they feel uncomfortable. This is because they have been using positions and techniques designed for people with high levels of flexibility and the majority of people are not very flexible.. Some of the stretching positions we have used traditionally are now known to be injurious. For example, the "hurdler's position" puts the knee in a position of misalignment which can cause injury to tendons and ligaments. The good news is that a regular stretching program can produce results, be painless, and promote relaxation and release of muscle tension. Chapter Three details contraindicated stretches and gives alternatives for safely increasing flexibility.

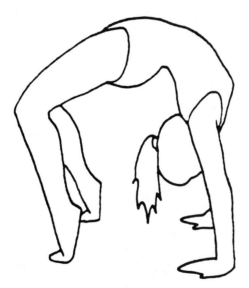

A gymnast performing a back arch. This high degree of flexibility is not necessary to function normally in every day life and may be injurious to someone who is not properly trained.

Body Composition

Your body weight includes the weight of all your muscles, bones, organs, body fluids and body fat. If the fat is removed, all that remains is your *lean body mass*. Exercise works to increase the lean body mass and decrease the body fat.

Your percentage of body fat is a much better indicator of your fitness than your weight. For example, the majority of football players would be obese according to typical weight charts. However, if we measured their percentage of body fat, it would probably be within normal ranges. To the contrary, there are many thin, sedentary people who weigh very little but are obese according to their body fat. It would be dangerous for these individuals to lose weight, they must exercise to increase their lean muscle mass.

Long-term regular exercise usually decreases body fat but does not have an immediate effect on body weight. This is because you are gaining muscle mass as you lose the fat. If you are trying to lose excess weight, do not become discouraged if your weight does not change immediately. Remember that your body composition is improving. Because lean tissue is more metabolically active than fat, you will burn more calories all of the time, even when you are sitting around or sleeping! Exercise also increases your ability to mobilize and oxidize fat. This enhances weight loss efforts, conserving lean body mass and preventing regain of lost body weight.

Average body fat ranges somewhere between 18% to 25% for females and 15% to 20% for males. Women are considered to be trim at 18-22%, men at 12-15%. Women are considered to be obese at a body fat over 30%, men over 25%. There are no proven ill effects for males who achieve extremely low body fat percentages. Some male distance runners have body fat levels as low as 4%. Females who drop below 12% to 15% may cease menstruating, although the cause is unknown. The decreased estrogen level promotes calcium loss from the bones, increasing the risk of osteoporosis. This is a common problem for long distance runners and other endurance athletes. To the contrary, high body fat is associated with cardiovascular disease, diabetes and some cancers so it is crucial to maintain a healthy body composition level.

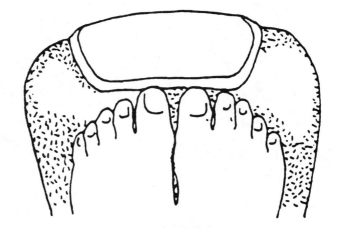

Scales may not give us all of the information needed to determine health status. The body fat percentage is often more important.

There are several methods for measuring body fat. A trained professional can determine your skinfold measurements by using calipers which measure the thickness of your skin at various sites. These measurements are used to estimate your percentage of body fat. Underwater weighing is another effective technique but requires expensive, cumbersome equipment and is often not practical. Looking objectively at your physique often tells you as much as you need to know without specific tests. It is important to remember that your body type and genetic background do play a part in determining your body composition. Decide what you can achieve realistically and slowly work toward your goal.

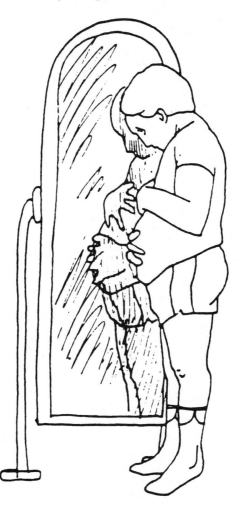

Americans are bombarded with advertisements, television programs and movies which show beautiful people with perfect physiques. Our genetic makeup plays a large role in what our bodies look like so it is important to remember that you are what you are and you can only change so much. You can, however, make the most of what you have. Exercise, proper nutrition, and a positive body image will help you to achieve your goals.

Notes

Chapter Two

THE BENEFITS OF EXERCISE

Hundreds of scientific and practical experiments have been carried out in an attempt to pinpoint the benefits of regular exercise. Some of the information is conflicting but overall the data suggests that being fit can have a positive impact on many aspects of your life. The list below highlights some of the well accepted benefits of exercise. Most of the benefits are related to aerobic exercise, however, people who lift weights or who are generally active will experience some of the same results. Recent studies have demonstrated that moderate activity is just as beneficial as strenuous, high-intensity exercise in preventing heart disease and increasing longevity. You don't have to run marathons to receive the benefits. Modest amounts of physical activity, such as climbing stairs, gardening, and walking the golf course, will have a positive impact on health.

Physiological Benefits of Regular Aerobic Exercise

1. Lower Resting Heart Rate - This means your heart has to beat fewer times per minute to supply your body with adequate oxygen and nutrients.

2. Lower Weight and Body Fat - Since obesity is a major risk factor for cardiovascular disease, diabetes and other health problems, reducing your risk could save your life. Lean body mass (muscle) is more metabolically active than fat which means you will burn more calories at rest.

3. Reduced High Blood Pressure - Exercise has been found to decrease elevated systolic and diastolic blood pressure.

4.   Decreased Blood Triglycerides and Cholesterol - Exercise has been shown to effectively reduce triglycerides, total cholesterol and LDL cholesterol all of which are related to a higher incidence of coronary artery disease (blockage of arteries which can lead to chest pain and/or heart attack). HDL cholesterol, a beneficial type of cholesterol which helps clear the arteries, is usually increased. Therefore, regular aerobic exercise combined with a low-fat/high-fiber diet can reduce the buildup of the plaque which causes blockage in arteries.

5. Higher Maximal Oxygen Uptake - Since your heart can pump more blood per beat, your body's capacity to consume oxygen during exercise is enhanced. The greater volume of blood (and therefore oxygen) delivered to the muscle cells results in increased stamina.

6. Increased Muscular Strength and Elasticity - As we grow older strength and flexibility become a deciding factor in our ability to function in normal and necessary activities. Exercise has been shown to delay and possibly prevent some of the degenerative problems associated with aging.

7. Enhanced Bone Health - Weight-bearing exercise such as recreational jogging, aerobic dancing, brisk walking and cycling can increase skeletal mass. Inactivity, on the other hand, contributes to calcium loss from the bones and to osteoporosis. Regular weight-bearing activity begun at an early age combined with proper nutrition can have a positive effect on lifelong bone health.

8. Decreased Incidence of Heart Disease - Major studies also show that if regular exercisers do have a heart attack they have less chance of a fatal or recurring event.

9. Longer Lifespan - Several studies indicate that people who are more active in every day activities and/or exercise regularly live longer than sedentary individuals.

Psychological Benefits of Regular Exercise

1.   Reduces Depression

2.   Improves Confidence and Self-Esteem

3. Promotes a Sense of Well-Being

4. Improves Ability to Handle Stress

5.   Decreases Tension

6. Improves Attitude Toward Work

7. Improves Overall Quality of Life

Chapter Three

WARMING UP FOR A
SAFE WORKOUT

Both competitive and recreational athletes often make the mistake of equating the words "warm-up" and "stretching." Although stretching exercises should be included in the pre-workout routine, the most important goal when preparing to exercise should be to increase the body temperature and to prepare the muscles, connective tissue, and circulatory system to safely accommodate more intense exercise. Stretching cold can be more harmful than not stretching at all.

For these reasons the warm-up phase is divided into two parts: The *circulatory warm-up* followed by the *stretching warm-up*.

The Circulatory Warm-up

The circulatory warm-up should be designed to raise local and core temperature and to increase blood flow to the working muscles. Because of this increase in temperature and blood saturation, a proper warm-up improves performance and reduces injury. Improved blood flow is necessary so that enough oxygen and nutrients are carried to the cells and so that the additional waste products produced can be adequately removed. The heart also has time to adjust to the increased demand. The higher body temperature allows nerve impulses to travel faster which maximizes coordination. In addition, the metabolic reactions that produce fuel for activity occur more quickly and more efficiently. In the muscle, the mechanical efficiency of contraction is enhanced and the contraction itself is quicker and more forceful. Muscles are more elastic and the extensibility of tendons, ligaments and other connective tissue is increased.

These physiologic principles make a strong case for not omitting the circulatory warm-up. It is especially important when exercise is performed in a cool or cold environment. Extremely cold surroundings may require a ten to fifteen minute circulatory warm-up.

Practically, the circulatory warm-up is simple. Performing medium intensity, general movements for four to six minutes will accomplish the intended goal. If an active warm-up is not possible or convenient, a passive warm-up such as a hot shower or applied heat can also be effective. Examples of proper circulatory warm-ups include:

Walking with arm movements
Slow cycling, swimming or jogging
Mild rope skipping
Low intensity aerobic dance routine

Remember that no stretching should be included during this segment. The circulatory warm-up should continue until a very light perspiration is present. At this point you should not feel tired or out of breath. Your heart rate and respiration rate are slightly elevated, your muscles are warmer and you are ready to proceed to the next portion of your workout.

Stretching Warm-up

Three to five minutes of mild stretching exercises should follow the circulatory warm-up. The purpose is to prepare your body for the stress of exercise. Stretching prevents injury by relaxing contracted muscles and lengthening tendons and connective tissue. The muscles are still not as warm as they should be, therefore, more intense stretching is better left for the end of the workout. Warm tissues stretch more easily, providing more permanent results and less risk of injury. A good rule to follow is: **Stretch first to prevent injury, stretch last to increase or maintain flexibility.**

Final Stretch

The final stretch is the last segment of your workout and should consist of five to ten minutes of stretching and relaxation exercises. Since your muscles are completely warm, it is okay to stretch with more intensity than you did in the stretching warm-up. In addition to increasing or maintaining flexibility, this last segment serves as a final cool-down from the aerobic and muscular conditioning exercises. After the final stretch you should feel slightly fatigued but not exhausted. Your body temperature and heart rate should be close to your resting levels and the majority of perspiration should have evaporated.

Types of Stretching

There are three basic types of stretching.

Ballistic stretching consists of quick, repetitive, bouncing type movements. Although this method is somewhat effective, the increased range of motion is achieved through a series of jerks and pulls on the resistant muscle tissue. The momentum can result in damage to muscle and connective tissue and may be responsible for increased muscle soreness.

Static stretching involves going into a position of stretch until tension is felt. The position is then held for ten to thirty seconds or even longer. Since static stretching is more controlled, there is less chance of exceeding the limits of the tissue thereby creating injury.

Contract and Relax methods involve contraction of muscles or muscle groups for five to ten seconds followed by relaxing and stretching. Traditionally, this procedure has been utilized by therapists for rehabilitation purposes. If carefully instructed and supervised, contract/relax methods can be effective in flexibility programs. Some of the positions require a partner, however, which increases the risk of overstretching and consequent injury.

General Rules for Stretching Safely

Avoid Hyperextension of the Spine - This arched position places the back in an extremely vulnerable position. The same compression that occurs with forward flexion also makes arching the back dangerous.

Avoid Locking any Joint - When stretching, performing muscular conditioning exercises, lifting weights or any other activity it is important to keep the knees and other joints "softened" to guard against unnecessary stretching or tearing of ligaments and connective tissue.

Never Force a Movement - Do not place your body in unnatural positions and do not perform movements which cause discomfort. Listen to signals that you may be overextending your limits.

Avoid Forward Flexion of the Spine - Some of the positions which result in a high injury rate involve forward flexion of the spine. Forward flexion simply means bending forward from the waist.

The spine is a flexible column formed of a series of bones called vertebrae. The vertebrae are stacked on top of each other with the spinal cord running through the middle. Between each one are intervertebral discs which are filled with a soft, pulpy, highly elastic substance. These discs act as cushions for the bony vertebrae, however, they tend to degenerate with age, sometimes beginning as early as age 25. Forward flexion causes the front border of the intervertebral discs to compress. The pressure this places on the pulpy center can be so great that it ruptures causing severe back pain. The problem is magnified if any twisting motion is added to the forward flexion (windmills, side bends, elbow to knee, etc.). Over time these positions contribute to chronic degeneration and can greatly increase the chance of low back pain or herniation of a disc.

This position also forces the hamstrings to stretch and contract simultaneously in order to maintain balance. The muscle cannot relax and thus the stretch will be less effective. In addition, too much time in this inverted position may cause an adverse blood pressure response.

When lifting heavy objects we are often reminded to use our legs, not our back. The justification for this is the same as for avoiding forward and side bending exercise positions. Exercise is not the only culprit. Gardening, tying your shoes, and other forward bending movements can all contribute to wear and tear on the discs.

CONTRAINDICATED STRETCHING POSITIONS: WHAT TO DO INSTEAD

The positions described in this chapter are frequently used as stretching exercises. They are divided into muscle groups and are then catagorized as "contraindicated," "conditional," or "safe." Read this section and then use *The Five Minute Stretch* (Appendix 1) to begin your flexibility program. It is a summary of the safe positions and includes all major muscle groups.

CONTRAINDICATED

It is best to completely avoid *contraindicated* positions or stretches. Although it is not guaranteed that an injury will result, the chances are much increased and there are always safe and effective alternatives. Even if you do not feel pain while performing a contraindicated stretch, damage may be occurring which will show up later in life.

CONDITIONAL

Some positions are not really dangerous, they are just uncomfortable and ineffective for individuals who have poor flexibility in a specific joint. These are called *conditional* exercises and should only be used if they feel comfortable and if they accomplish the desired goal for each individual.

SAFE

Safe positions can be used by almost everyone but precautions still need to be taken to assure correct form and technique.

Stretching the Neck and Shoulders

Never Hyperextend the neck
This means you should not bend your neck to the back or do full head circles. This compresses the cervical discs and can result in acute or chronic injury.

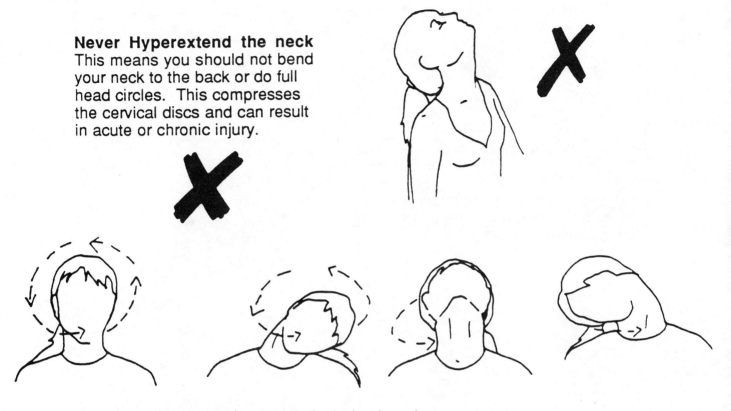

Slow, static stretches which include dropping the head to the center, turning to each side, and placing the ear to the shoulder will safely relieve tension and tightness in the neck and shoulders.

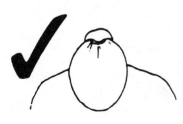

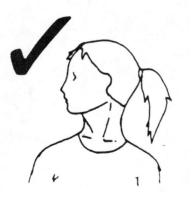

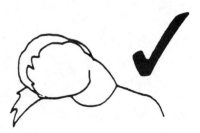

17

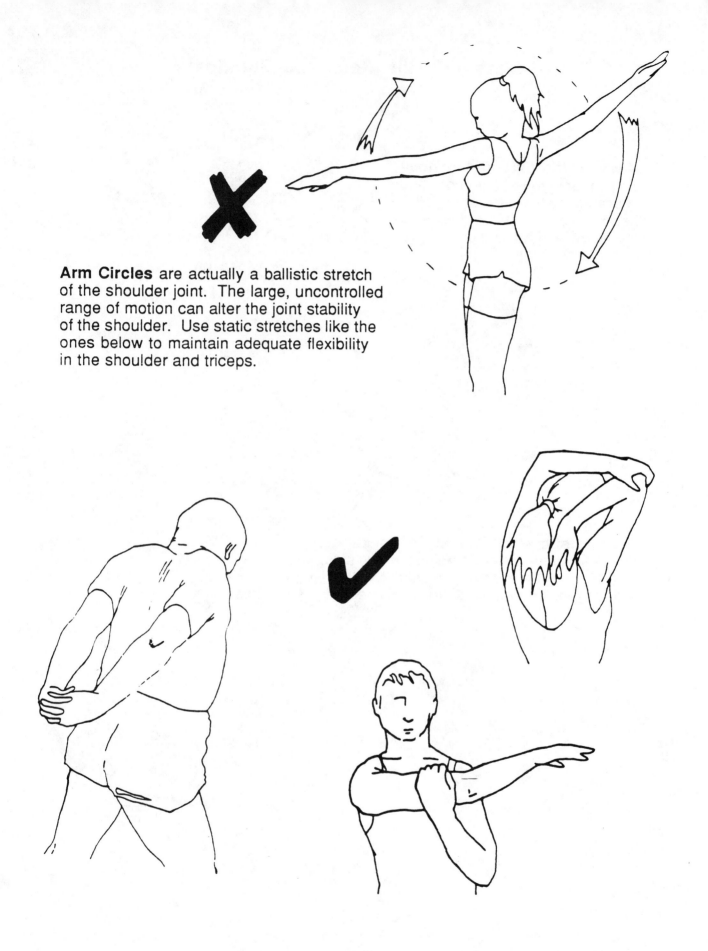

Arm Circles are actually a ballistic stretch of the shoulder joint. The large, uncontrolled range of motion can alter the joint stability of the shoulder. Use static stretches like the ones below to maintain adequate flexibility in the shoulder and triceps.

Stretching the Upper Body and Torso

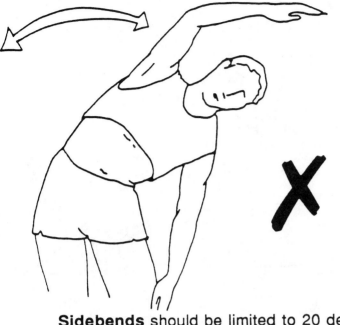

Sidebends should be limited to 20 degrees in order to prevent compression of the vertebral discs. You can stretch the same muscles by simply reaching in an upward direction with one arm. The knees should be bent and the buttocks tucked under to keep the spine in a straight line.

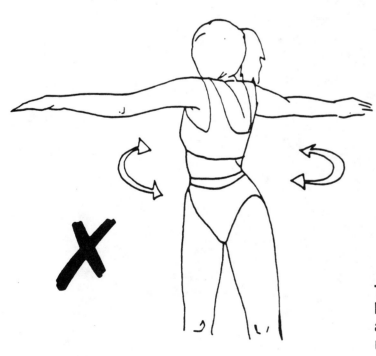

Twisting movements are ballistic in nature and should be avoided. They are likely to result in injury to the vertebral discs.

19

Stretching the Lower Back

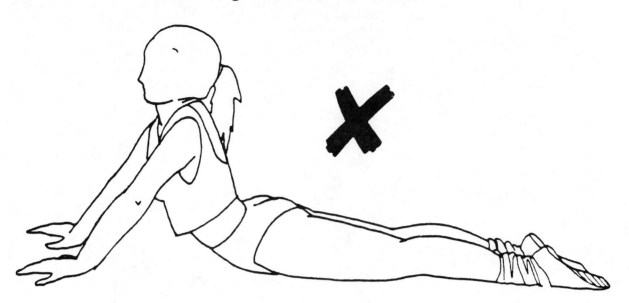

Never hyperextend the back - Arching the back while stretching or exercising is likely to cause injury due to compression of the spine and misalignment.

The plow position compresses the cervical vertebrae of the neck and puts a large amount of stress on the lower back. Avoid this exercise completely.

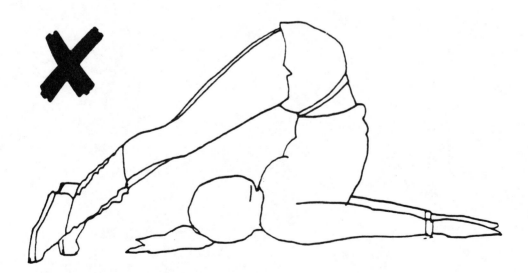

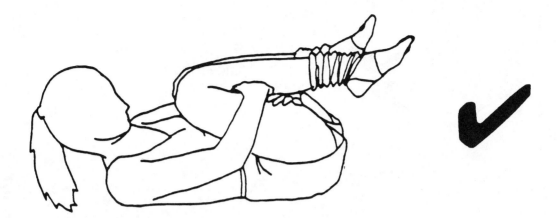

To safely stretch the lower back, pull your knees to your chest, hold beneath your knee caps (to prevent overbending of the knee joint), and curl up in a ball. Hold this position for at least 10 seconds.

Another excellent stretch for the lower back involves lying on the back with one knee to the chest. Keep the other foot on the floor and press your lower back into the floor.

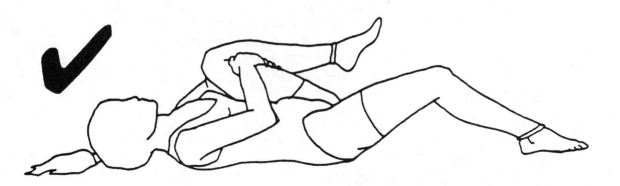

Stretching the Quadriceps

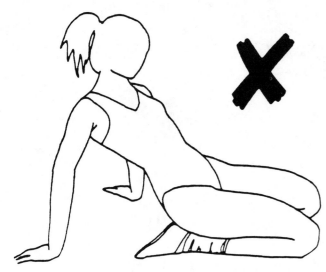

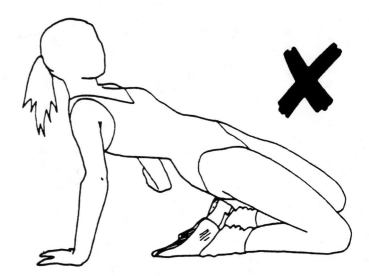

This stretch overbends the knee joint and places the back in a hyperextended position.

It is okay to use this stretch if you are able to comfortably and correctly maintain this position. The knee should never lean over the toe as this places too much weight and force on the joint. Keep the back straight and lower the hips toward the floor until you feel the stretch.

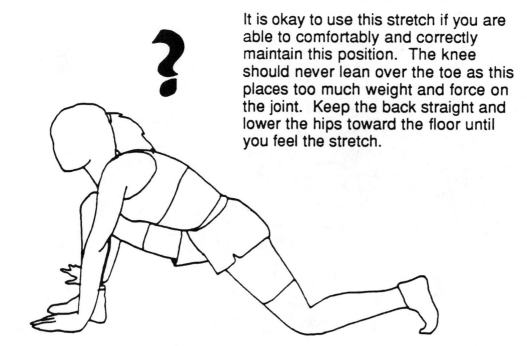

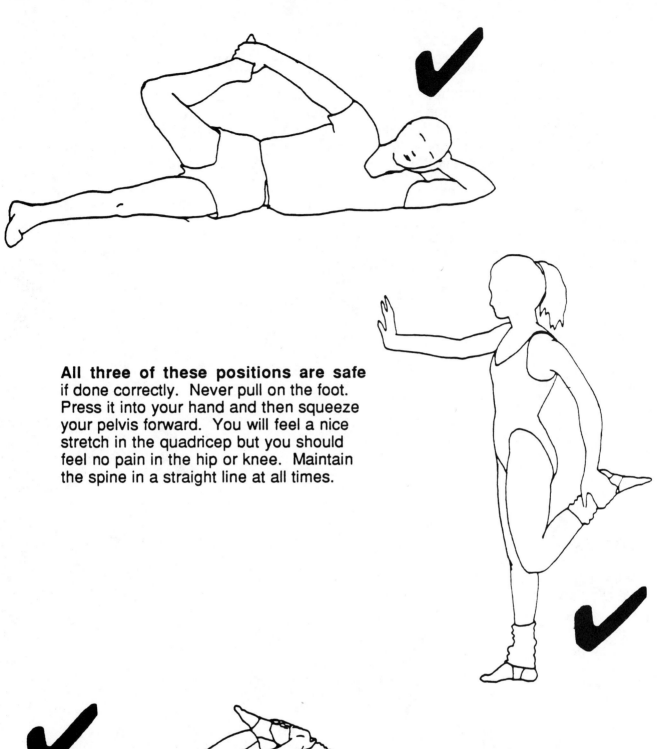

All three of these positions are safe if done correctly. Never pull on the foot. Press it into your hand and then squeeze your pelvis forward. You will feel a nice stretch in the quadricep but you should feel no pain in the hip or knee. Maintain the spine in a straight line at all times.

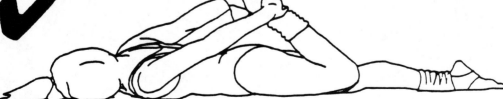

Stretching the Hamstrings

All six of the stretches on this page involve forward flexion of the spine and thus are contraindicated. Many are traditional positions that we have always done so it is difficult to remove them from your workout. Just remember that there are many safe and effective alternatives that could prevent lower back pain and other problems in the future.

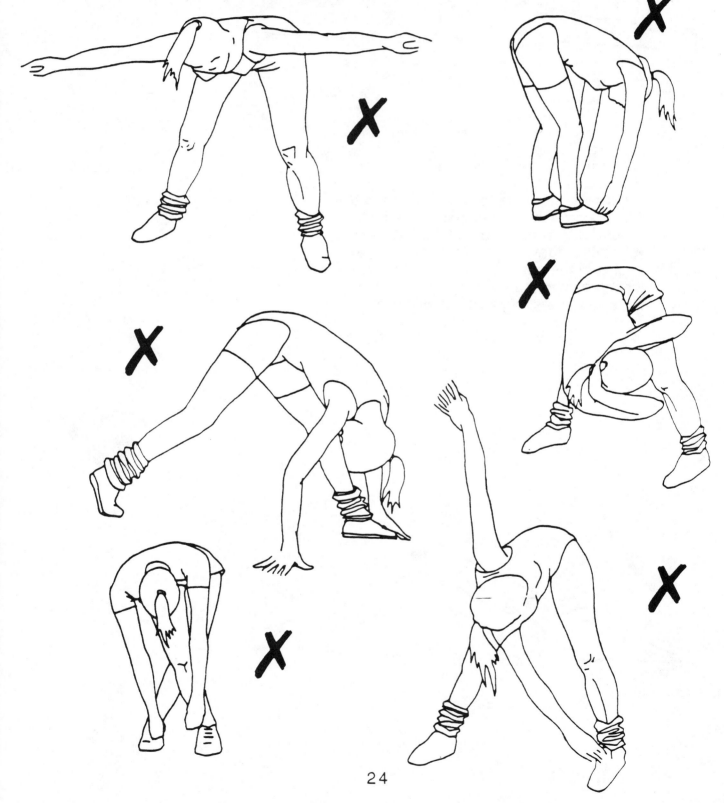

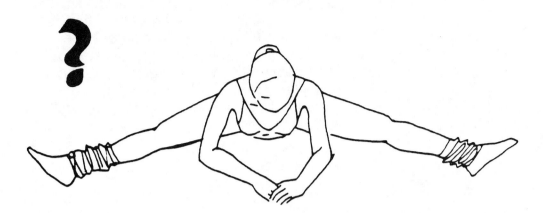

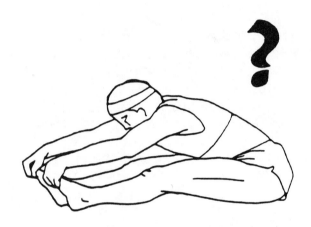

Sitting toe touches and straddle
stretches are safe if and only if
you are flexible enough to keep
your spine in a straight line.
There are more comfortable
ways to stretch the hamstrings
if this one causes you discomfort.
If you prefer these positions,
make sure you keep your knees
soft and only go forward to the
point of tension.

This hamstring and adductor
stretch is contraindicated because
bending to the side places the spine in
a position of misalignment. Never
bend more than 20 degrees to the
side.

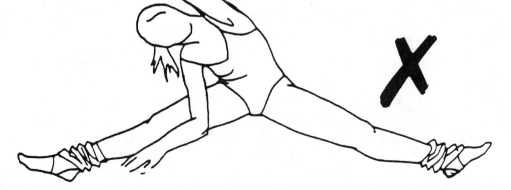

The safest way to increase flexibility in the hamstrings is on the back with one foot flat on the floor and the other knee pulled to your chest. Hold beneath your knee cap and slowly straighten your knee until you feel tension in the hamstring (never lock the knee). Hold for a minimum of 10 seconds.

This modified position is much safer than the traditional "hurdler's stretch" which places stress on the ligaments and tendons in the knee. When performing the modified hurdler keep the knee soft, the spine straight, and only go forward until you feel tension. If you feel the stretch sitting straight up, then hold that position. Don't worry if you can't go very far.

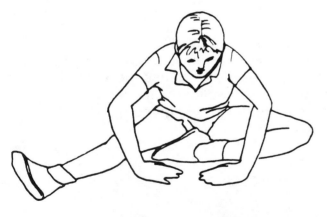

It may be more convenient or comfortable to stand up to stretch. Just place your foot on a low step or bench, keep the knee bent, and bend from the hips until you feel the stretch.

Stretching the Adductors

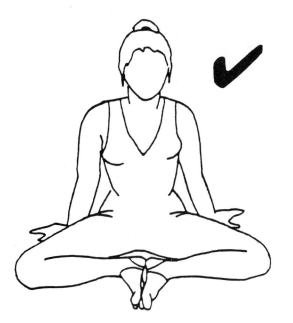

Safely stretch the adductors by sitting with the soles of the feet together and the arms supporting the back. Gently press the knees down and hold. This same stretch works well lying down as the floor supports the back.

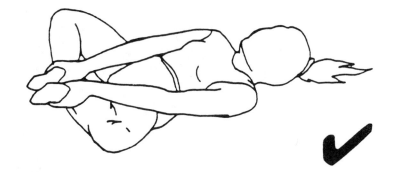

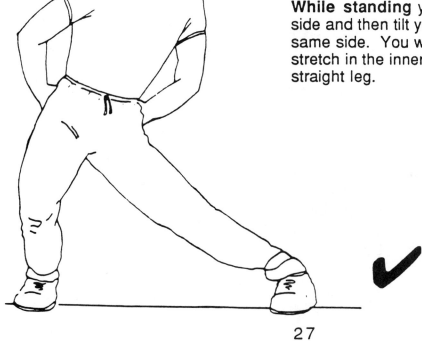

While standing you can lunge to one side and then tilt your hips to that same side. You will experience a mild stretch in the inner thigh of your straight leg.

Stretching the Gastrocnemius

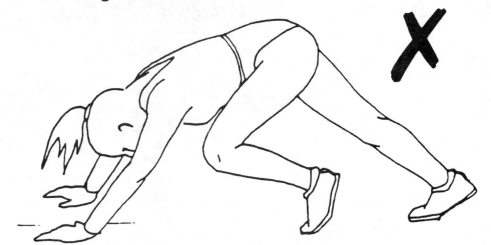

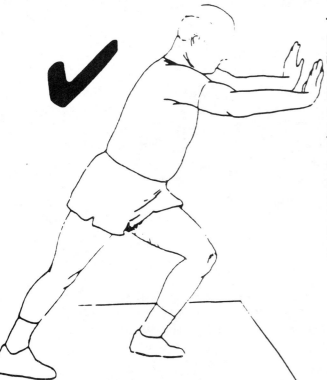

The position above relies on a hand support position which may inhibit blood from flowing back to the heart. The low head position may also initiate an adverse blood pressure response. Simple flexion of the ankle joint will gently stretch the calf muscle. Another popular and effective stretch involves pushing against a wall or solid object. Be sure to keep the spine aligned at all times. To help prevent shin splints it is also important to stretch the tibialis anterior on the front of the lower leg.

Chapter Four

AEROBIC EXERCISE

Taking part in regular aerobic exercise will help you achieve cardiovascular health and will promote a feeling of physical and mental well-being. Contrary to the marketing claims of fad diets and exercise gimmicks, aerobic activity is the only way to effectively burn body fat. The good news is that it does not have to be difficult or painful to achieve these benefits. Although it is best to follow the guidelines of intensity, frequency, and duration outlined in this chapter, any safe activity is better than nothing. So start moving!

Choosing an Aerobic Activity

There are many aerobic activities from which to choose. The decision should be based on your preferences, your present and past health and the equipment and facilities you have available to you. The activities below can all be considered aerobic. They are divided into low-impact and high-impact. Low-impact activities are not necessarily lower intensity. In fact, higher impact activities such as running and high level aerobic dance are associated with certain musculoskeletal injuries because of the vertical forces on the joints. One advantage of high-impact activity is that the weight-bearing exercise helps to maintain or increase bone mass. This may help prevent osteoporosis. If you choose a high-impact activity, make sure you have the proper shoes and a safe surface on which to exercise. It may be helpful to alternate low-impact with high-impact workouts. For example, running alternated with swimming. This is called "cross-training" and helps to reduce boredom as well as injury. People with health considerations such as knee or back problems should always choose a low-impact type of exercise. Others simply find that low-impact is more enjoyable. The key is moderation. You should be able to continue regular exercise for your entire life. Starting out with a fun, safe program and progressing gradually will increase your chances of sticking with an exercise program.

Low-Impact Activities	**High-Impact Activities**
Walking/Hiking	Jogging
Aqua-Walking/Aqua-Jogging	Running
Swimming	High-Impact Aerobic Dance
Stationary Biking	Rope Skipping
Road Cycling	
Low-Impact Aerobic Dance	
Bench-Step Aerobics	
Aqua Aerobics	
Rowing	
Cross Country Skiing	
Stair Climbing	

This is not a complete list. Any activity which meets the requirements of frequency, duration, and intensity will achieve the desired results.

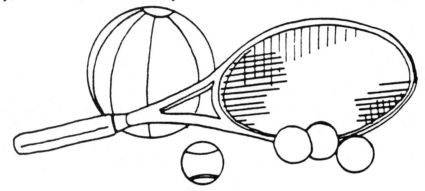

Sports such as tennis, racquetball and basketball are sometimes considered aerobic, however, there are often too many stops and starts to maintain the necessary heart rate. They still burn calories, reduce stress, and provide some aerobic benefit.

Frequency, Duration & Intensity of Aerobic Exercise
Based on Guidelines from the American College of Sports Medicine

Frequency
Research has demonstrated that significant gains in cardiovascular endurance can result with a minimum of three non-consecutive days of aerobic exercise per week. Unless you wish to train for a marathon or other athletic event, three days a week is plenty to improve your health and fitness. If weight control is a priority, however, exercising aerobically four to seven days a week will burn more calories. In this case extreme caution is necessary in order to avoid overuse injuries.

Duration
To achieve gains in cardiovascular endurance it is necessary to raise the heart rate into the target zone and maintain it for at least 20 minutes. Up to 60

minutes is acceptable, however, the longer you exercise the greater the chance of injury. Progression is very important so start with 5 or 10 minutes in your target zone and add a few minutes with each workout until you reach your goal.

Always finish your aerobic activity with at least 5 minutes of walking or low-level activity. If you stand still while your heart rate is elevated, the blood will pool in your legs and you may become faint or dizzy. Keep moving so the muscles can pump blood back up to your heart. When your heart rate falls below 120 beats/minute it is usually safe to stop.

Jogging is a popular aerobic activity.

Intensity

The intensity of an aerobic exercise session is best measured by the exercising heart rate. The proper heart rate range is called the "Target Heart Zone" and is based on your age and resting heart rate. The intensity should also be based on factors such as previous exercise experience and current fitness level. For most healthy people, a range somewhere between 60% and 90% of their estimated maximal heart rate is best. If you have never exercised before, you should start with a lower intensity level and progress gradually. Beginners should work closer to 60%, intermediate level individuals can work at 75% to 80%, and advanced or competitive participants can work at 90%.

Research has shown that in order for cardiovascular training effects to occur, one has to exceed the lower level of the target zone during aerobic exercise. Equally important is the higher portion of the target zone. When your heart rate exceeds this level, you may be working at an intensity so high that your *aerobic* (with oxygen) energy system cannot meet the body's demand for oxygen. At this point your *anaerobic* (without oxygen) system begins to produce much of the energy used. Although both aerobic and anaerobic exercise burn calories and increase endurance, overweight individuals are better off working at a lower intensity for a longer duration. Also, for some individuals it can be dangerous to exercise at a very high intensity. Some medications for high blood pressure and other problems increase or decrease the heart rate. In this

31

case intensity cannot be measured by monitoring the heart rate and a physician should be consulted to determine the correct mode and level of exercise.

Monitoring Your Pulse

Heart rates should be taken once before, twice during, and once after the aerobic segment of your workout. When you first begin an exercise program it may be necessary to take it more often. Take your pulse either on the thumbside of your wrist (radial pulse) or the groove in your neck (carotid pulse). Make sure you use your first two fingers and not your thumb. Your thumb has its own pulse and may cause you to count inaccurately. Count for 6 seconds and multiply by 10 or simply add a zero. For example, if your pulse beats 15 times in 6 seconds, your heart rate is 150. It helps to practice taking your pulse so you can do it quickly and accurately when exercising. Since, your heart rate during exercise is related to how you feel, after a while you will be able to tell when you are working at the correct intensity. This is called your "perceived exertion" and is an accurate and accepted method of monitoring intensity.

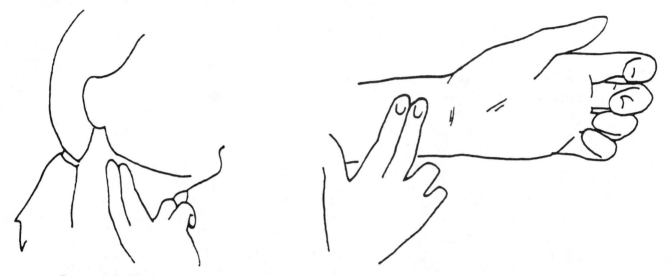

Carotid Pulse   **Radial Pulse**

Determining Your Resting Pulse Rate

Immediately after awakening from a good night's sleep lay very still and find your pulse. Count it for a full minute. This is your resting pulse rate. Use it in the equation on the next page to calculate your Target Heart Zone. If you have not been exercising regularly you can expect your resting heart rate to decrease as you become more fit. This means your heart will pump more oxygenated blood to your body with fewer beats.

Calculating Your Target Heart Zone

Follow the equation (The Karvonen formula) on the next page to determine your individual target zone. In step three you can change the intensity to accomodate your fitness level. Beginners should multiply by .65, intermediate exercisers should multiply by .75, and trained athletes should use

.85. This equation may not be appropriate for elite athletes. Their cardiovascular systems are so efficient that they cannot raise their heart rates high enough. This does not mean they are not benefitting from the aerobic activity. If you do not know your resting heart rate use the chart on page 36 for a Target Heart Zone based only on age. If you are on medications that lower or raise heart rate (i.e. beta blockers) you cannot use heart rate as an accurate measure of intensity. Consult with your physician.

The Karvonen Formula

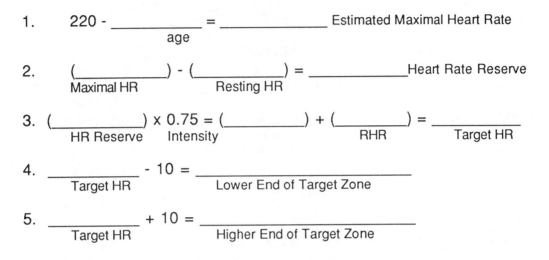

1.   220 - _____ = _____ Estimated Maximal Heart Rate
              age

2.   (_____) - (_____) = _____Heart Rate Reserve
    Maximal HR   Resting HR

3.   (_____) x 0.75 = (_____) + (_____) = _____
    HR Reserve   Intensity   RHR   Target HR

4.   _____ - 10 = _____
    Target HR   Lower End of Target Zone

5.   _____ + 10 = _____
    Target HR   Higher End of Target Zone

Example
A 45 year old female wants to determine her Target Heart Zone. She takes her pulse upon awakening and finds it to be 69 beats per minute.

1. 220 - 45 (age) = 175 (Estimated Maximal Heart Rate)

2. 175 (MHR) - 69 (Resting HR) = 106 (Heart Rate Reserve)

3. 106 (HRR) x 0.70 (Intensity) = 79.5 +69 (RHR) = 148.5 (Target HR)

4. 149 (Target HR) - 10 =   **139** (Lower End of Target Zone)

5. 149(Target HR) + 10 =   **159** (Higher End of Target Zone)

She should maintain a pulse of <u>139 to 159</u> throughout her 20-30 minutes of aerobic exercise (14 to 16 beats in six seconds).

The Bell Curve Concept

Use the "bell curve" technique for designing your aerobic workout. Start out slowly (at the bottom of your THZ). Slowly increase the intensity and keep your heart rate near the top of your THZ for 10 to 15 minutes. Taper down at the end so when you complete a total of 20 to 30 minutes you are back down to the lower level of your target zone. Always finish with a low-intensity cool-down to bring your heart rate below 120 beats/minute.

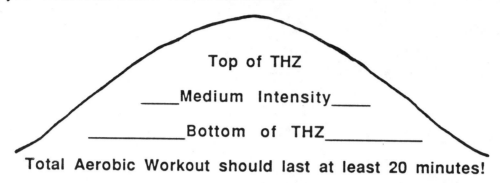

Top of THZ

_____Medium Intensity_____

_____Bottom of THZ_____

Total Aerobic Workout should last at least 20 minutes!

Safety Tips for Common Aerobic Activities

Aerobic Dance

The crucial ingredient for a safe and effective class is a trained and concerned instructor. Check qualifications and background before you begin the class. Other important features include a proper surface such as a wooden floor or a specially designed aerobic floor, a controlled environment that is not too hot or too cold and appropriate, well-fitting footwear. Recent studies indicate that the arm movements in aerobic dance may produce a higher heart rate than other activities even though the intensity (oxygen consumption) is the same. Don't worry if you stay at the top of your Target Heart Zone as long as you can talk normally and feel okay.

Walking

Many people are choosing a walking program to achieve aerobic benefits. The advantages are numerous. You can walk anywhere, it costs very little money and you can continue for a lifetime of safe exercise. Sometimes it is difficult to bring the heart rate into the target zone but this can be facilitated with light hand weights and/or a very rapid pace. Ankle weights are discouraged because they increase the force of impact on the feet and joints. Proper shoes are also imperative to prevent injury.

Jogging

Jogging is an important part of the lifestyle of literally millions of people. It is an effective way to increase fitness and health, it requires very little equipment and you can do it almost anywhere. Proper shoes are a must. If you are a new jogger go to a reputable dealer who can help you choose a running shoe to serve your individual needs. If you have been jogging take your old shoes with you. A knowledgable salesperson can tell a lot about your biomechanical style by the wear patterns on your shoes. Replace your shoes as soon as they wear out to guard against stress injuries.

There is no one correct way to jog but some simple guidelines may prevent an injury. Stand erect and keep the spine as straight as possible. Your arms should be relaxed and bent at the elbow. They should swing front to back with no side to side motion. The most important factor is the way your foot makes contact with the running surface. Land on the back third of your foot, roll forward and lift from the front of your foot to push forward for the next step. The running surface is also a potential source of chronic injury. Smooth, even surfaces are best. Cement and concrete are very hard and thus result in more injuries than grass or track surfaces.

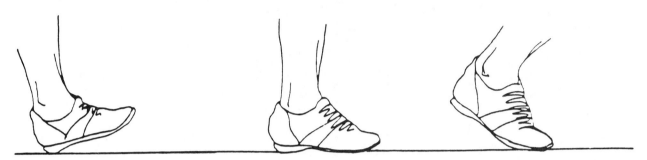

The proper foot strike sequence when running or jogging.

Swimming
This activity is perfect for almost everyone, but especially those with orthopedic problems, joint discomfort, pregnant women, the elderly, obese or overweight individuals and many others. The water supports the weight of your body so there are few overuse or impact problems. To assure your safety make sure you are comfortable in the water and that there are lifeguards available at all times. Cleanliness and proper maintenance of the pool facility are also important.

Cycling
Progress slowly, walking and other aerobic activities will not prepare your leg and thigh muscles for intense cycling. If cycling along roads, wear appropriate safety equipment (i.e. helmet and reflective materials) and observe proper rules and regulations of the road. Stationary biking is great for winter months and rainy days, however, do not invest in expensive equipment until you have proven you will stick with it. Walk for several months and then reward yourself with a stationary cycle.

Cross-Training
You can achieve the same or greater cardiovascular endurance level by varying your aerobic activities This helps prevent boredom and decreases overuse injuries. For example, walking Monday, Wednesday, and Friday and cycling on Tuesday and Thursday.

Target Heart Zone

Based on Age
70% TO 85% OF MAXIMUM HEART RATE

AGE	70%	85%	AGE	70%	85%
15	144	174	47	121	147
16	143	173	48	120	146
17	142	173	49	120	145
18	141	172	50	119	145
19	141	171	51	118	144
20	140	170	52	118	143
21	139	169	53	117	142
22	139	168	54	116	141
23	138	167	55	116	140
24	137	167	56	115	139
25	137	166	57	114	139
26	136	165	58	113	138
27	135	164	59	113	137
28	134	163	60	112	136
29	134	162	61	111	135
30	133	162	62	111	134
31	132	161	63	110	133
32	132	160	64	109	133
33	131	159	65	108	132
34	130	158	66	108	131
35	130	157	67	107	130
36	129	156	68	106	129
37	128	156	69	106	128
38	127	155	70	105	128
39	127	154	71	104	127
40	126	153	72	104	126
41	125	152	73	103	125
42	124	151	74	102	124
43	124	150	75	102	123
44	123	150	76	101	122
45	123	149	77	100	122
46	122	148	78	99	121

Chapter Five

MUSCULAR STRENGTH AND ENDURANCE

This portion of the workout can last anywhere from ten to sixty minutes depending on the time, space and equipment available. It normally follows the aerobic section but can be done on alternate days or immediately after the warm-up.

The Concept of Overload

If a muscle, muscle group or the cardiovascular system is worked harder than it is normally accustomed, it will eventually improve and become more efficient. As one level becomes less demanding you can work slightly harder the next time and you will continue to improve. This concept applies to aerobic exercise as well as to weight training and calisthenics.

The Spot Reducing Myth

Body fat cannot be altered by specific spot reduction exercises. The burning of body fat during exercise follows a biologically selective pattern with the least stable fat deposits being utilized first. Calisthenics and weight training exercises work to build and tone muscle while burning virtually no fat. Body fat is a primary energy source only when exercising aerobically within your target heart zone. The amount of fat burned will depend on the duration and intensity of your workout.

Muscular Strength Development

The key to significant strength increases is the amount of tension produced by a muscle. The way to improve muscular strength is to perform exercises that require few repetitions but involve large amounts of tension. The best method of accomplishing significant strength gains is through weight training. Weight training for strength will produce significant hypertrophy (increased muscle size) in the male because of the hormone testosterone.

Females need not worry about becoming muscle bound since they do not have high levels of testosterone.

Significant strength gains can also be achieved by adding resistance to regular exercises. For example, abdominal curls with weights in the hands or upper body work with stretchy bands. Consult your physician prior to lifting weights or using stretchy bands if you have high blood pressure, are pregnant, have Carpal Tunnel Syndrome, or any other injury or condition that could limit physical activity.

Muscular Endurance Development

By overloading the muscles so that their need for oxygen is increased, the ability to continue sustained and repeated contractions is enhanced. This is accomplished by working the muscles frequently and by using high numbers of repetitions. Weight training and stretchy bands as well as numerous calisthenic exercises will increase muscular endurance.

A combination of strength training and endurance training is optimal for achieving benefits related to health. Increased strength in the appropriate muscle groups will help correct muscle imbalances. Increased endurance will result in better muscle tone and an improved ability to carry out daily tasks.

Alternatives for Building Strength and Endurance

Calisthenics: Abdominal curl-ups, modified and regular push-ups, side leg lifts, tricep lifts, etc. require no special equipment and can greatly enhance muscular conditioning. Mats or a carpeted area are necessary for proper cushioning. In an outdoor area a towel can be placed on the grass.

Weight Training: If weight training equipment is available the following prescription should be used for those trying to increase overall strength, endurance and muscle balance: Since there is a large variety of equipment, make sure you are oriented and instructed as to proper use of the equipment and proper technique.

Rubberized Resistance: Many people do not have convenient access to weight training equipment or facilities. Studies have demonstrated that adding resistance to our muscle work greatly enhances muscular strength. Exercising with rubberized resistance such as the DYNA-BANDS® shown in this chapter is a quick, convenient way to build muscular strength and endurance at home, at work, on vacation, or anywhere There are several brands of rubber bands that can be used to increase strength and endurance. Some, like the DYNA-BAND come in different levels of resistance. Old car or bicycle inner tubes can be cut into strips and washed to serve the same purpose.

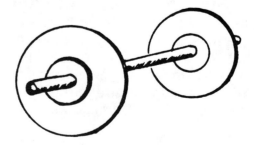

The following prescription should be used to increase overall strength, endurance and muscle balance: The American College of Sports Medicine recommends at least two non-consecutive days per week.

1-2 Sets of 8 to 12 repetitions with weights or bands
Light to moderate weight or resistance - Choose a weight such that you feel the fatigue on the last 3-4 repetitions.
Proper Progression - Begin at 8 repetitions, work up to 12, and then increase the weight slightly and go back to 8 repetitions.
Proper Body Position - If any position or exercise causes discomfort it should be discontinued immediately. The back and the knee are most vulnerable to injury so avoid locking the knee and never hyperextend (arch) the lower back while lifting weights.

For Muscle Balance:
Abdominals
Hamstrings
Rhomboids (Upper Back)
Triceps
Abductors (Outer Thighs)

For Additional Toning and Strengthening:
Pectorals (Chest)
Biceps
Adductors (Inner Thighs)
Gastrocnemius (Calves)
Quadriceps

Safety Tips for Weight Training and Muscle Work
Never perform muscle work without completing a circulatory and stretching warm-up.

Never lock the knees or elbows during any exercise. Maintain enough control so that you straighten the joint without snapping it.

The highest priority should be to avoid hyperextending the neck, the back, or the knees. Keep your spine in alignment at all times.

Deep knee bends or squats should be avoided. They place too much stress on the knees and back.

Avoid exercises which involve forward flexion of the spine (for example, bent over rows).

Working the Upper Body

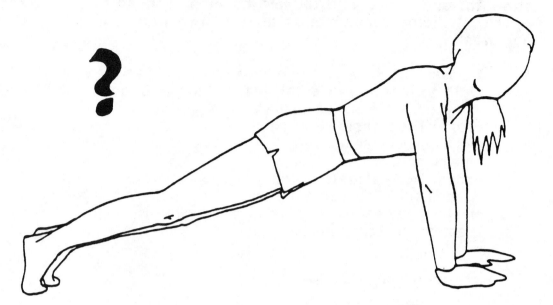

When performing push-ups make sure you are strong enough to keep your spine in line. The back should not arch and the buttocks should not raise to dip the chin. When you approach the "up" position do not snap your elbows into a locked position. Modified push-ups do not require as much strength as regular push-ups and allow better control of body position.

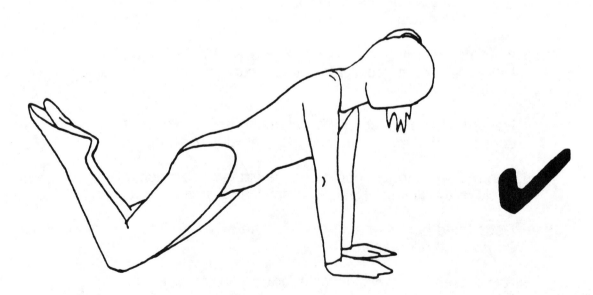

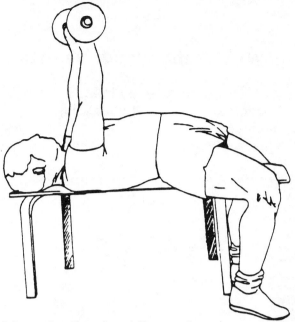

Avoid arching the back while performing any weight training exercise on a bench. Putting your feet on the bench with the knees bent will protect your lower back. Also remember to control each movement so that you never snap or lock a joint.

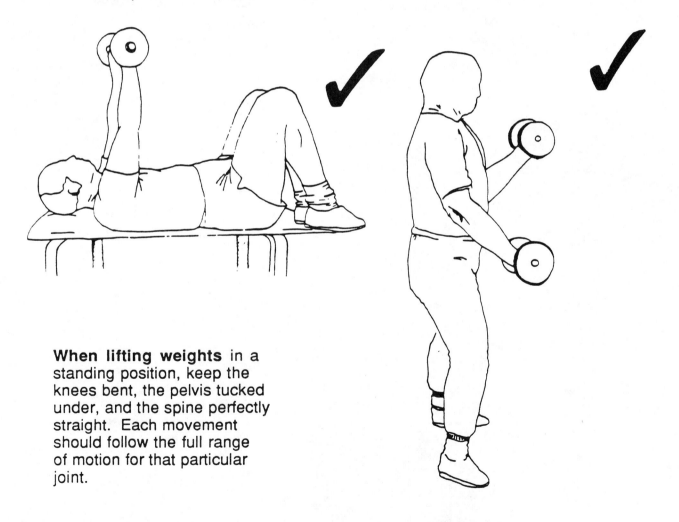

When lifting weights in a standing position, keep the knees bent, the pelvis tucked under, and the spine perfectly straight. Each movement should follow the full range of motion for that particular joint.

Exercising With Rubberized Resistance

Safety Tips: Bend your knees on all exercises.
Do not hyperextend or lock your joints.
Never hold your breath. Exhale on the hardest portion.
Control every movement. No bouncing or jerking.

There are limitless exercises that can be performed with the DYNA-BAND®. Here are six that you can do in ten minutes to get a well-rounded upper body workout.

Pectorals/Chest

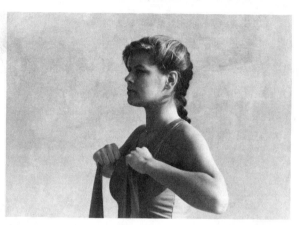

Starting Position
Wrap band behind your back. Grab each side close to your underarms. Bend knees.

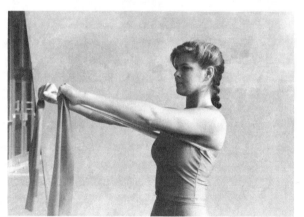

Contraction
Extend straight out. Exhale as you extend. Inhale as you return to the starting position.

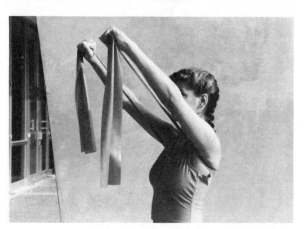

Variation
Extend at a 45 degree angle.

Upper Back/Chest

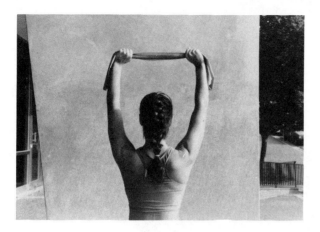

Starting Position
Hold band above your head with hands about eight inches apart. Bend knees. Tuck pelvis under.

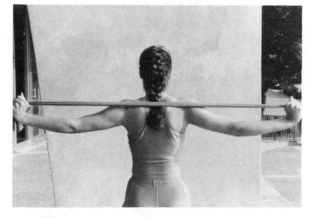

Contraction
Pull out and down behind your head, bringing shoulder blades together. Do not arch the lower back. Return to the starting position.

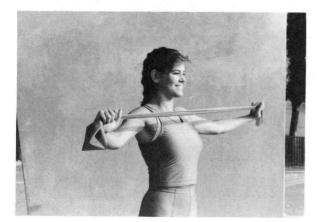

Variation
Pull out and down to the front. Return to the starting position.

Biceps

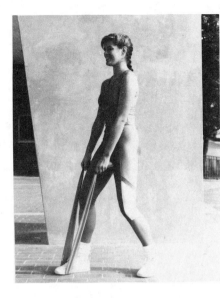 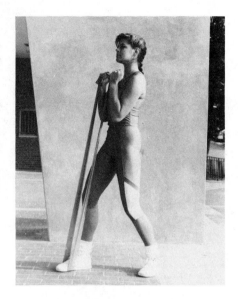

Starting Position
Bend knees. Place center of band under one foot and grab each end.

Contraction
Slowly curl. The only motion is from the elbow down.

Deltoids

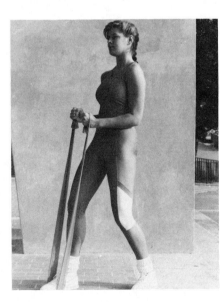 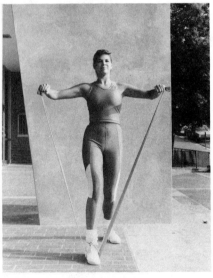

Starting Position
Bend knees. Place center of band under one foot. Grab band and wrap over the top of each hand.

Contraction
Lift arms as a unit, leading with the elbows. Do not lift higher than shoulder level.

44

Triceps

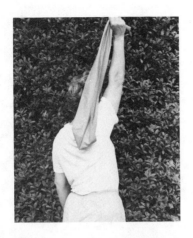

Starting Position
Bend knees. Hold band in your right hand with your arm by your ear.

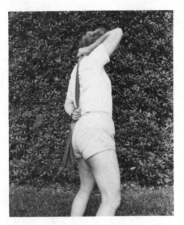

Stabilization
Bend elbow and grab with the left hand behind the back.

Contraction
Stabilize the left hand and slowly extend the right arm. Repeat on the other side.

Triceps (alternative)

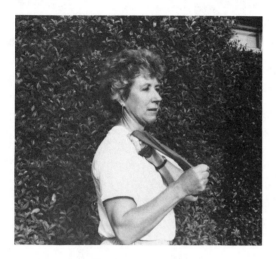

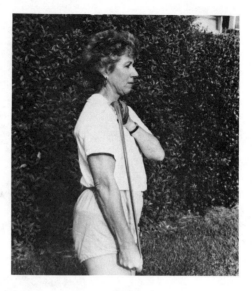

Starting Position
Wrap band around your left hand and place on the right shoulder. Grab with the right hand.

Contraction
Extend the right arm down along your side. Repeat on the other side.

Shoulder Shrugs

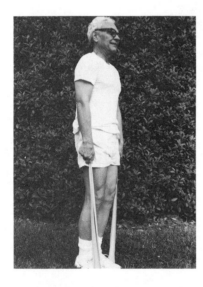

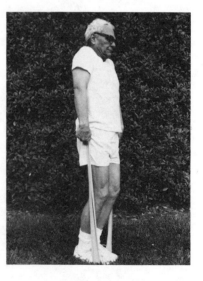

Starting Position
Stand on center of band with both feet. Grab each end. Bend knees.

Contraction
Lift and lower the shoulders. Also try forward and backward shoulder rolls.

Working the Abdominals

The abdominals include the rectus abdominus, the transverse abdominus and the internal and external obliques. Traditionally, full sit-ups, elbow to knee positions, and straight leg lifts have been the preferred exercises for strengthening the abdominals. The problem is that these exercises actually contract the hip flexors (iliopsoas) which are already strong. This cheats the weaker abdominal group and increases the degree of muscle imbalance. Once you curl your torso up past 30 degrees the hip flexors take over. This is why you feel your legs tighten as you do a full sit-up. To prevent this problem, pull your heels as close to your body as possible or cross your legs straight in the air. You will not be able to come up as far but now you are isolating your abdominals and making them do all the work.

Go slowly and control each curl-up. Exhale as you curl up and inhale as you lower. Come up as far as you can without tightening your thighs. This will insure that you increase abdominal strength through the full range of movement.

Avoid full sit-ups with the hands behind the head. When you become fatigued it is tempting to pull on your head in order to complete the sit-up which may result in cervical vertebrae damage. The straight-leg position places great strain on the lower back. By placing your feet under a bar you are allowing the hip flexors to do even more of the work.

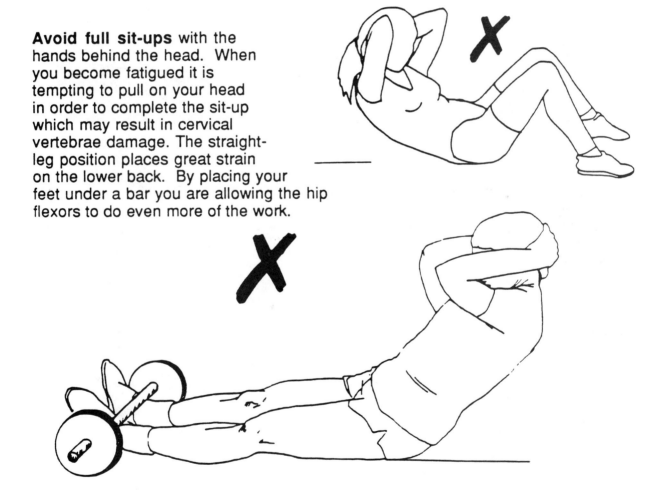

Avoid elbow to knee exercises. They primarily work the hip flexors and place strain on the neck and spine. The "six inches off the floor" exercise is extremely dangerous. It places tremendous strain on the lower back and depends almost totally on the hip flexors.

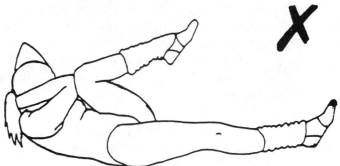

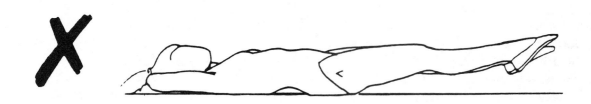

Curl ups in these positions are safe and effective. The leg position prohibits the hip flexors from contracting, therefore, allowing the abdominals to do most of the work. Arms can be crossed on the chest, touching the ear lobes or shoulders, or you can perfom chest presses or bicep curls as you do the abdominal work.

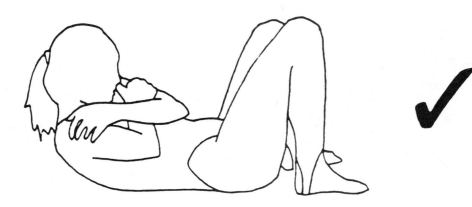

Slowly lift and lower your buttocks to perform reverse sit-ups. This is an effective alternative or addition to the curl-ups above. You can also do a combination curl-up and reverse sit-up. Simply curl-up with the hands on the shoulders as you simultaneously lift the buttocks. Slowly release and repeat.

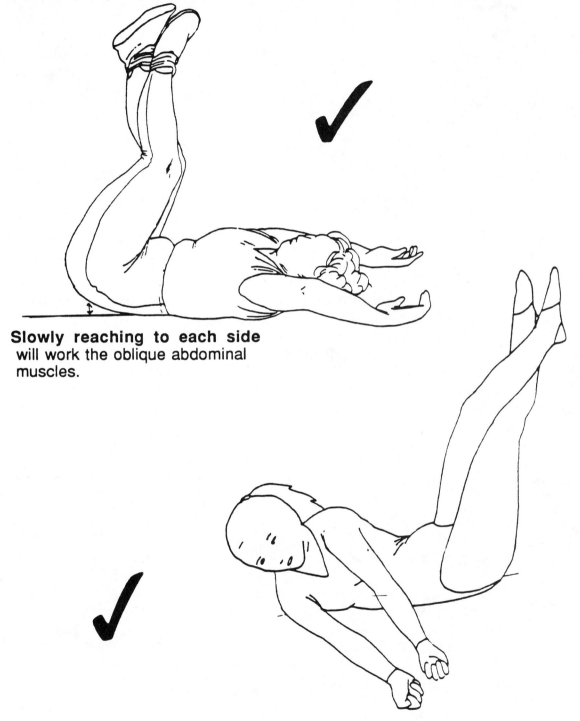

Slowly reaching to each side will work the oblique abdominal muscles.

Hip and Thigh Work

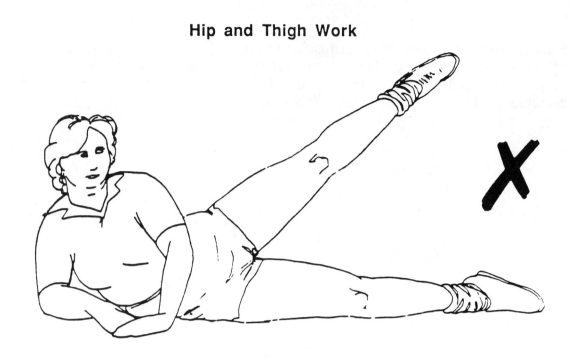

The side lying position can be used to work the abductors, adductors, and gluteals. You should not be up on your elbow because it compresses the vertebral discs. The knee and toe should point forward so that the hip does not move out of line with the shoulder. Protect the lower back from arching by pulling the bottom knee forward. The top knee should remain slightly bent.

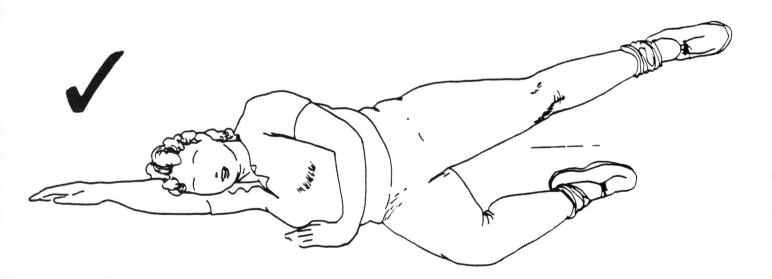

Hamstrings

To strengthen the hamstring, hold on to a sturdy object and pull the heel toward the buttocks. It is not necessary to come all the way up, just to a comfortable angle. Keep the support leg bent and the spine straight. Do enough repetitions to achieve overload or add ankle weights.

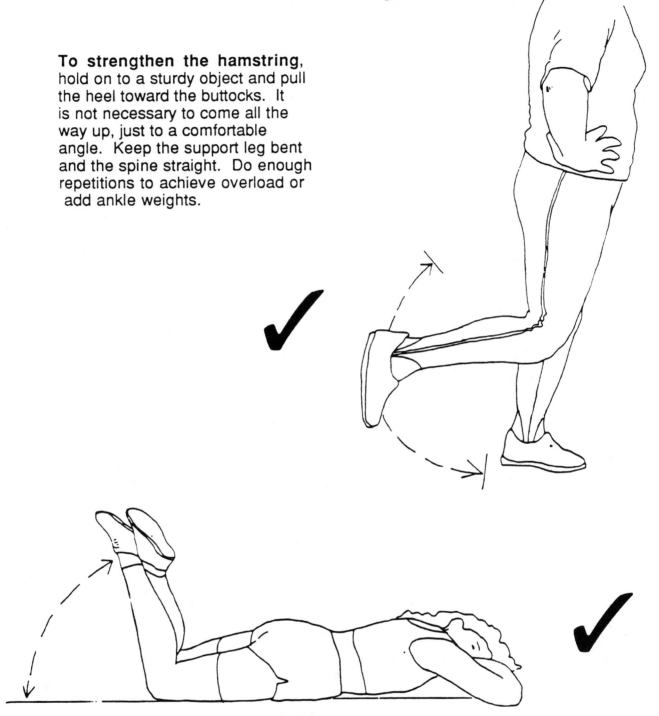

This exercise is excellent because it provides added resistance. Lie prone with the ankles crossed. Slowly pull the bottom foot toward the buttocks while resisting with the top foot. Do the reverse as you return to the starting position.

Muscles and Muscle Groups

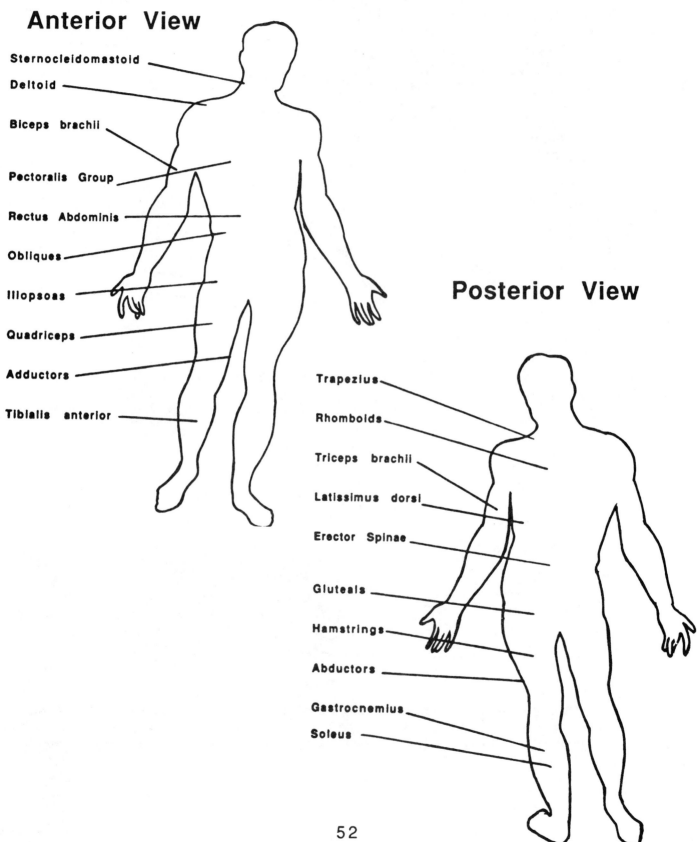

Anterior View

- Sternocleidomastoid
- Deltoid
- Biceps brachii
- Pectoralis Group
- Rectus Abdominis
- Obliques
- Iliopsoas
- Quadriceps
- Adductors
- Tibialis anterior

Posterior View

- Trapezius
- Rhomboids
- Triceps brachii
- Latissimus dorsi
- Erector Spinae
- Gluteals
- Hamstrings
- Abductors
- Gastrocnemius
- Soleus

Chapter Six

EXERCISE FOR SPECIAL POPULATIONS

Arthritis

The two basic forms of arthritis, *osteoarthritis and rheumatoid arthritis*, have different causes but both result in pain within the joints. This pain leads to limited use and therefore decreased range of motion. A longer warm-up is essential for arthritic patients in order to enhance joint mobility.

The best form of aerobic activity is swimming or aqua-aerobics which both reduce impact stress on the joints. It may be necessary to decrease intensity and duration and to increase frequency. Strength building, slow, static stretching and range of motion exercises should also be a priority. Hand or leg weights should not be used.

Remember to progress slowly, discontinue any exercise which causes discomfort and consult your physician if you experience any severe pain.

Cardiovascular Disease

Persons with diagnosed cardiovascular disease can benefit greatly from rehabilitative exercise programs. These programs should only be conducted by qualified medical personnel with emergency equipment readily available. Often, after a patient has progressed successfully, a physician will give clearance for exercising outside the program. To maximize safety and to minimize a recurring cardiovascular event, patients should proceed very gradually, never exercise alone and get specific recommendations from the physician with regard to frequency, intensity and duration. Check to see whether any prescribed medications affect normal heart rate response to exercise. Patients should also be alert for symptoms such as shortness of breath, chest pain, dizziness or any other sign of discomfort.

Diabetes Mellitus

Physical exercise has been found to have an insulin-like effect on the body and thus facilitates the entry of glucose into the cells. Exercise is appropriate only when performed under a physician's guidance and in combination with dietary and/or medical controls.

Simple carbohydrates, such as candy, fruit juice or sugar should be readily available at the exercise site in case hypoglycemia develops. Diabetics who use insulin should avoid injections into muscles which will be used directly in their workout.

Specific exercise plans will depend on each individual's health and fitness status as well as the advice of their doctor.

Hypertension

Persons with high blood pressure should always obtain medical clearance before performing any type of exercise. A low to moderate intensity aerobic activity is best. Information about how the patient's medication will affect the heart rate should be provided by the physician. Hypertensive exercisers should avoid any static or isometric contractions which can raise blood pressure to dangerous levels. For example, straining to lift a heavy weight or pushing against a stationary object. Also, activities which require raised arm positions for long periods can increase pressure. In addition, an extended warm-up, cool-down and relaxation segment will increase the safety of the workout.

Overweight or Obese Individuals

A person should be judged obese by evaluation of both body fat percentage and body weight. Since movement and balance are limited to some degree, exercise is more difficult. Low-impact aerobic dance, walking, swimming, aqua-aerobics or riding a stationary bicycle are all appropriate choices. Intensity should be set at 55% to 70% of maximal heart rate reserve. Duration and frequency should be increased to facilitate weight loss (30-50 minutes, 4-7 times/week). A serious weight loss program will include exercise and moderate dietary restrictions. The maximal rate for safe weight loss is 1-2 lbs per week. Patience and diligence will eventually pay off where fad diets and rubber suits will result in large swings of weight loss and weight gain. Recent research indicates that this yo yo type of dieting may permanently lower metabolism making it harder and harder to lose the weight that is regained.

Pregnancy

With proper supervision, exercise for the pregnant woman can be extremely beneficial. The purpose is to maintain aerobic fitness and muscle tone, to prepare for labor and delivery and to increase self-esteem and emotional health. Activities like swimming, aqua-aerobics and stationary cycling are excellent. The American College of Obstetricians and Gynecologists has determined guidelines and recommendations for exercising during the pregnancy and during the postpartum period. These guidelines can be obtained from your obstetrician who can also advise you on your individual status.

54

Chapter Seven

NUTRITION FOR AN ACTIVE LIFESTYLE

A healthy diet enhances the benefits gained through regular exercise. Aerobic workouts combined with proper nutrition will aid in weight control, help reduce calcium loss from bones and help reduce stress and anxiety. No matter what your personal goals for wellness are, a nutrition plan will be beneficial. The good news is that you don't have to drastically change your lifestyle or go on one boring, impossible diet after the other. A few carefully made changes can modify your nutritional habits for a lifetime of healthy eating.

The Balance Equation for Weight Control

The term *weight control* means to attain or maintain your optimum body weight through a combination of regular exercise and balanced nutrition. This includes gaining weight, losing weight or staying where you are. The basic principle of weight control is simple. Your energy intake (food) and your energy output (physical activity) must be kept in balance. If you start to gain a few pounds you simply increase your daily activity and/or decrease what you consume each day.

Most people attempt to lose weight by counting calories which are actually kilocalories (kcals). A kilocalorie is a unit of energy which is used as fuel for your metabolic and physical activities. Energy can come in the form of fat, carbohydrate, protein or alcohol. If your goal is weight loss, you should attempt to use up calories stored as fat by burning off more calories than you take in. It takes about 3500 calories to make one pound of fat so you must burn 3500 excess calories to lose one pound of body weight.

ENERGY INTAKE = ENERGY OUTPUT
(food)   (metabolism and physical activity)

Remember that the number of calories you need will vary depending on many factors. Bodysize, metabolic rate, severe illness or injury, pregnancy, lactation or other conditons can all influence energy requirements.

Dieting is Out
Research has recently demonstrated that we have been trying to lose weight the wrong way for hundreds of years. Every time we go through the lose-gain-lose-gain cycle we are permanently lowering our metabolism, making it even harder to lose the next time. Try making small changes that you can stick with forever. Slow, gradual weight loss (1-2 lbs/week) achieved by increasing activity and replacing fat and sugar with complex carbohydrates is the key to success.

The Essential Nutrients

Carbohydrates
55% or more of the calories in your total diet should be composed of complex carbohydrates. Foods such as cereals, fruits, vegetables, rice, bread and pasta are good choices. Traditionally people have believed that eating these "starchy" foods would contribute to weight gain, however, when eaten unrefined, they satisfy the appetite, provide large amounts of vitamins, minerals, and fiber and are relatively low in calories.

Refined or simple sugars are also carbohydrates but are not as nutritionally beneficial as the complex carbohydrates. Most foods which contain a lot of sugar are "empty calories". They are completely devoid of essential nutrients but contain a high number of calories. Consuming large amounts of sugar has been linked to severe dental caries as well as chronic diseases such as heart disease, diabetes and obesity.

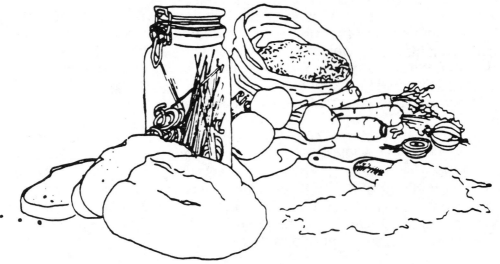

Fats
No more than 30% of your caloric intake should come from fats. The majority of the fat you take in should be composed of unsaturated fats from vegetable sources. Animal fats tend to higher than vegetable sources in

saturated fatty acids and cholesterol. The best fats to use for cooking are olive oil, canola oil, or other mono- or poly-unsaturated fats.

Some common foods which should be severely limited are high-fat dairy products, luncheon meats, fried foods and butter. Some foods, especially animal products (meats, eggs, cream), are very high in cholesterol. Cholesterol is not a fat, it is a lipoprotein which is only found in animal products. High levels of cholesterol in the bloodstream are related to increased risk for coronary artery disease. High-fat diets in general are related to cardiovascular disease, cancers of the bowel and breast, gall bladder disease and obesity. Lowering your intake of high-cholesterol and high-fat foods as well as performing regular aerobic exercise are the best ways to decrease your risk and to control your weight.

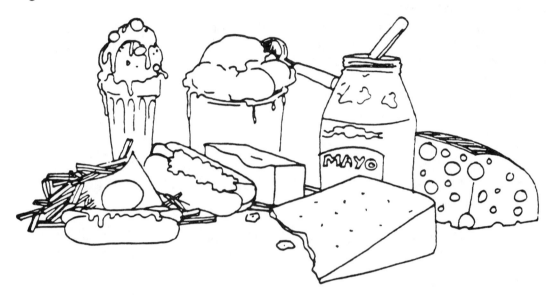

Protein
Protein is required as a source of essential amino acids and nitrogen. 15% of your diet should be composed of low fat protein such as chicken, fish, lean beef, and vegetable sources. Americans tend to consume vast amounts of unneeded protein. High protein diets result in no special advantage and may actually be harmful. Depressed growth rates in rats, toxic effects in premature infants, increased calcium loss in adults and progressive renal dysfunction have all been linked to high protein diets. Certain conditions such as adolescence, pregnancy, lactation and illness may require higher than normal protein intake. Try eating more beans, grains, and low-fat dairy products (like skim milk and yogurt) to get your daily protein requirement.

Vitamins
Vitamins include 13 different organic molecules which are not synthesized in adequate amounts within the human body. A well- rounded diet should provide all the nutrients necessary for optimal health.

Minerals and Trace Elements

Minerals are essential substances that are widely available in food but are present in small amounts. Calcium and Iron are the minerals most likely to be deficient, especially in females.

Water

Adequate water intake is necessary to replace fluids lost through vigorous exercise. The amount lost depends on many factors including environmental temperature, humidity and your ability to dissipate heat. Drink water before, during and after your workout.

Be a Smart Consumer

Shopping is one of the hardest parts of eating a healthy diet. Labels and advertisements are deceptive. The following tips will help you spend your money wisely.

Any diet or plan that claims large decreases in weight in a short amount of time should be avoided.

Cholesterol is not a fat. If the label says "no cholesterol" it can still be 100% fat. Cholesterol is only found in animal products, thus foods like peanut butter and margarine will never have cholesterol but are very high in fat calories.

Avoid foods made with palm, palm kernal, or coconut oil. These are highly saturated fats which can raise blood cholesterol and triglycerides.

The following terms all mean one thing - sugar! No one sugar is healthier or better than another. *Brown sugar, honey, dextrose, maltose, lactose, fructose, rock sugar,* and *corn syrup* (fructose may be absorbed slower which is beneficial for some diabetics).

Look at the list of ingredients on a label. The first on the list is the most abundant in the food. Therefore if *dextrose* is listed first, you know the food is mostly sugar.

Check serving sizes. Most of us eat much more than a typical serving.

Protein, fat and carbohydrate are listed by weight, not percentage of total calories. This can be very deceiving since fat has more than twice the calories per gram than protein or carbohydrate. In the example below, milk that is 2% fat by weight is actually 38% fat by calories. You don't need to carry your calculator to the store when you shop. Just be aware of the amount of fat in the foods you normally purchase. Make substitutions for the high fat foods.

Reading Labels

1 gram of fat	=	9 kilocalories
1 gram of protein	=	4 kilocalories
1 gram of carbohydrate	=	4 kilocalories
1 gram of alcohol	=	7 kilocalories

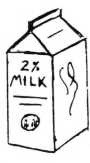

Example: 2% Milk

1 serving (1 cup) = 120 total calories

5 grams of fat X 9 calories = 45 calories from fat

45(fat) divided by120(total) = <u>38%</u> of calories from fat

If you choose non-fat or low-fat foods you get to eat over twice as much for the same number of calories! Try non-fat yogurt instead of sour cream on your baked potato, a whole plate of pasta instead of a hotdog, or two huge bowls of cereal for one sausage biscuit. Weight control is much easier because you are satisfied.

Ideas for Snacks

Fruits and vegetables are best!

Pretzels instead of chips and fried snacks

Air popped popcorn - if it's too dry try spraying with a butter flavored cooking spray and then sprinkle with parmesan cheese or other seasoning.

Make dip with non-fat yogurt or cottage cheese. Salsa or bean dip are also great choices.

Use cereal for a snack. Most are low in fat and make crunchy finger food.

Bagels, pita bread and low fat crackers are tasty and they fill you up!!

Other Nutritional Concerns

Alcohol
Alcoholic beverages are low in nutrient content and high in calories. For optimal health and weight control it is best to abstain or drink in moderation.

Supplements
If you eat a balanced, complete diet there is no need to take any vitamin or mineral supplements. Sometimes a deficiency, food allergy or other situation

requires the addition of nutrients to the diet. Females often do not get adequate calcium and/or iron in the food they take in, therfore, it may be necessary to take a supplement. Pregnant women, the elderly, the ill or injured, premature infants and teenagers sometimes need increased nutrients.

If you or your physician decide that you require a supplement, make sure that you do not consume more than the Recommended Daily Dietary Allowance for that particular vitamin or mineral. There are many *super vitamins* on the market which can cause health problems. Excessive amounts of Vitamins A, D, E, and K can be toxic.

Fiber

Fiber refers to the components of plant cell walls that are not digested by human intestinal enzymes. Fiber adds bulk to the diet, absorbs water in the intestine and produces larger, softer stools that are easily eliminated. The benefits of a high fiber diet include: lower rates of diverticulosis, colon cancer, and other digestive tract diseases; reduced serum cholesterol and serum glucose; and improved control of blood sugar and insulin levels in patients with diabetes mellitus. You can increase the fiber in your diet by eating more unprocessed foods such as fruits, vegetables and whole grains.

Sodium

Sodium is a mineral that occurs naturally in foods in combination with other chemical elements. It is also a nutrient that is essential for maintaining fluid balance and normal function of the heart and other muscles. The intake of sodium from all sources is usually much greater than the amount needed for normal growth, development and maintenance of health. Individuals with high blood pressure or strong family histories of hypertension should follow a diet low in sodium. Try to reduce the number of processed foods in your diet and limit the addition of table salt when cooking or seasoning your food.

Eating Disorders

With the emphasis in this country on beauty and possessing a perfect physique it is very difficult to maintain a healthy attitude concerning body image, eating, and weight control. Various eating disorders have become more prominant in recent years, especially among teenagers and young adults. Typically, but not exclusively, eating disorders are diagnosed in females of at least average intelligence but better than average achievement from middle to upper socioeconomic classes.

Anorexia Nervosa - This condition may include some or all of the following symptoms: a fear of obesity, disturbed body image, significant weight loss and refusal to maintain normal weight. Anorexics will honestly report feeling fat even though they are obviously emaciated. They usually remain highly active and deny interest in food. Many anorexics cease menstruating. There are other severe physical symptoms which result from this disease and in a percentage of cases death is the end result.

Bulimia - Bulimia is characterized by chronic binge eating. This involves rapid consumption of large amounts of food followed by large weight fluctuations, vomiting and/or abuse of laxatives and diuretics. Bulimics usually suffer from depression, feelings of shame, poor self-esteem and isolation. Bulimics are normally aware that their behavior is abnormal. There are several medical problems associated with binge/purge behavior such as gastric distention, poor diabetes control and clotting factor deficiencies. Dental erosion resulting from the hydrochloric acid in vomit is also a common symptom.

Bulimarexia - This term is used to describe those who exhibit symptoms of both bulimia and anorexia nervosa. For example, a chronic binge eater who purges and also has significant weight loss.

Treatment
The treatment of eating disorders is very controversial. Behavior modification, individual, group, or family therapy, diets, nutritional support and drug therapy have all proved successful in some cases.
The top priority is to attain professional medical help for victims of eating disorders.

Osteoporosis
Gradual bone loss is a consequence of aging. Osteoporosis is a condition marked by a loss of bone calcium and weakening of skeletal strength. The bones become so weak that the slightest trauma results in fracture. At highest risk is the white female who is relatively thin and sedentary. Black females are at lower risk probably because of greater bone mass. The cause of osteoporosis appears to involve several factors:

Lack of Exercise - Absence of weight-bearing exercise can result in a loss of bone calcium as well as a decreased ability to replace lost calcium. Recent studies indicate that weight training may be one of the most beneficial ways to build bone mass, along with activities like walking, jogging, rope skipping, and aerobic dance.

Postmenopausal Lack of Estrogen - The hormone estrogen is protective against excessive bone degeneration. This is one reason why physicians sometimes prescribe estrogen replacement therapy for women after menopause. Also at risk are premenopausal women who do not menstruate regularly for other reasons.

Lack of Vitamin C - Vitamin C is needed by bone-forming cells to make the structural support upon which bone minerals are deposited.

Lack of Calcium - If sufficient calcium is lacking in the diet it will be removed from bones to be used in other parts of the body. Try to consume adequate calcium in your diet but if this is not possible, supplements can be substituted. Some medical conditions, however, are compromised by calcium intake so check with your physician before taking high levels of calcium.

Notes

Chapter Eight

INJURY PREVENTION AND TREATMENT

The RICE Treatment for Fitness Injuries

REST -   Stop immediately when you feel pain.

ICE -   Apply ice for 24 to 48 hours (20 minutes on, 20-30 minutes off).

COMPRESSION -   Firmly wrap the injured area (not too tight) with elastic or compression bandages.

ELEVATION -   Raise the affected area to encourage blood flow to and from the injury.

In all cases, if pain becomes worse or persists for a prolonged period, seek medical attention immediately. Progress slowly upon resuming your activity.

Common Injuries Associated With Exercise

Muscle Soreness

Muscle soreness usually occurs when you begin an exercise regimen or you suddenly change the types of exercises you have been using. The key is prevention. Progress slowly! Start with low repetition and low intensity and make sure you warm-up and cool-down properly. Avoid ballistic movements and stretches. If you do become sore it will usually last 24 to 48 hours regardless of what you do to treat it. Sometimes repeating mild exercise the following day and then performing slow static stretches will relieve some of the discomfort. Massage and warm baths may also help.

Shin Splints

Inflammation or pain occurring where the muscles and tendons attach to bones can cause pain in the front portion of the lower leg. This can result from poorly fitted shoes, an improper running surface or a program which is too intense. An imbalance between the gastrocnemius and the tibialis anterior may also contribute to shin problems. Other causes of shin splints include: a lowered arch, irritated membranes, tearing of muscle where it attaches to bone, hairline or stress fracture of the bone or other factors. The best treatment is RICE, however, switching to a low impact activity for a while may allow time for healing while maintaining fitness.

Knee Problems

Pain in the knee can be very difficult to diagnose. Many times it is the result of overuse, poorly fitted shoes, improper running surfaces or biomechanical problems. Using proper progression, avoiding uneven surfaces and not allowing injuries to become chronic will help prevent serious knee problems. Always see a physician if pain persists.

Ankle Problems

Ankle sprains and twists often occur with activities that require quick changes of direction. Proper warm-up, taping or ankle supports and shoes with high support may help prevent ankle injuries. If an injury does occur the ankle should be iced immediately and medical treatment should be sought.

Achilles' Tendon

Achilles' tendonitis, which is inflammation of the sheath around the Achilles' tendon, can cause severe pain and is a frequent complaint of distance runners. Usually, improper shoes are the culprit and ice and rest are the treatment. In some cases surgery may be necessary.

Side Stitch

This is a sharp pain in the side beneath the ribs. Possible causes for this pain include: an oxygen deficiency, gas pains, spasms of the diaphragm or an improper warm-up. Often it will disappear if you lower the intensity of your activity, take slow, deep breaths, or bend toward the stitch and press gently on the painful area.

Heat Injuries

In extremely hot temperatures or high humidity you need to be very careful to avoid heat cramps, heat exhaustion and heat stroke. Heat cramps are the mildest heat-stress problem. Symptoms include muscle twitches and cramping in the arms, legs and abdomen. If you experience any of the following symptoms you may be suffering from heat exhaustion and should cool off and drink fluids containing potassium: headache, severe fatigue, nausea, low urinary output, clamminess, weak and rapid pulse, dizziness. Hot, dry, flushed skin, incoherent behavior, inability to perspire or seizures can be related to heat stroke and thus medical attention is required immediately. If not treated, heat stroke can be fatal.

Cardiovascular Problems

You should seek medical attention immediately if you experience any of the following symptoms while exercising or afterwards:

- Pain or pressure in the chest, the arm or the throat.

- Abnormal heart activity like fluttering, jumping or palpitations in the chest or throat.

- Nausea, dizziness, sudden lack of coordination, confusion, cold sweating, fainting or any other serious symptom

Lower Back Pain

It is estimated that over 80% of North Americans will experience back problems in their lifetimes. Our sedentary jobs and lifestyles are the primary cause. Most back injuries are the result of chronic degeneration over a long period of time. Poor posture, weak support muscles, inadequate flexibility, improper body mechanics, pregnancy and congenital problems can all lead to back pain or injury. There is no need to create a special exercise program for people with mild low back pain or injury. Everyone should follow a conservative, safe program such as the one in this book. Make sure you concentrate on strengthening the abdominals and hamstrings and delete any contraindicated exercises from your workout. Prevent back pain before it starts. Some lower back problems can be very serious and thus require immediate medical care. If in doubt, consult your physician.

Healthy Back Tips

When standing for long periods put one foot on a stool to prevent swayback.

When lifting, use a wide stance and bend the knees and hips, not the waist. Keep the object close to your body. Avoid twisting. If it is too heavy, get help!

Do not slump when sitting, pull abdominals in, keep spine straight and sit slightly forward.

If your chair is too high, swayback is increased. When sitting, knees should be even with the hips and feet should be flat on the floor.

Avoid leaning forward while sitting at a desk or table. If possible use a chair with armrests to reduce the load on your spine.

Wear comfortable shoes. Avoid high heels whenever possible.

The best sleeping positions are on the side with knees bent or on the back with a support under the knees.

Maintain ideal body weight.

Adhere to a regular exercise program.

Prevention is the Key

Progress slowly until a maintenance level is reached. Exercising too frequently or for long durations may predispose you to injuries. Never "work through the pain." If you feel any discomfort do not continue. Seek the appropriate treatment and do not resume the activity until the problem is corrected.

Chapter Nine

EXERCISE AND STRESS

Stress! We all have it. It can be positive or negative. However, too much of any stress can seriously affect physical and mental well being.

Good stress (eustress) offers opportunity for growth and satisfaction. Events such as starting school, getting married or achieving a promotion are eustressors. Distressors like financial problems, arguments and poor grades can be debilitating. Ability to manage stress can make an important difference in the quality of your life, and may actually influence your survival.

To deal with distress, first identify what it is that stresses you out. Is it at home, at work, with people, with family? Next, pinpoint your reaction to the stress. Physical responses like high blood pressure, insomnia, stomach disorders, ulcers, headaches, migraines and muscular tension can result. Withdrawing, crying, depression and other emotional responses are also common.

The next step is to remove or reduce the stress if possible. Sometimes the solution is as simple as summoning the courage to talk to someone about the problem and developing a compromise. Many times rearranging a room, changing a schedule or rotating responsibility will relieve stress. It is impossible to get rid of all of your stressors. Life would be very boring and not much of a challenge. Therefore, the final step is to learn to control the stress response and to minimize physical and mental reactions to everyday problems. This is where exercise can help.

Exercise and Stress Management

Exercise is one of the best ways to control and reduce the stress in your life. Activity provides a diversion, getting you away from the source of stress to clear your mind and to sort through the problem. Regular exercise makes you look better and feel better about yourself. Others will notice your improved self-concept.

Physiological changes that occur with long-term, regular activity provide more strength, endurance and energy to cope with difficult situations. Muscular tension which builds up throughout a stressful day is easily released with aerobic activity and stretching.

Exercise can reverse or improve many of the health problems that are related to stress. Benefits can include decreased high blood pressure, lowered cholesterol, improved sleeping patterns and lower body fat and body weight.

Stress Management Tools

Mental Imagery - During or after the final stretch of your workout clear your mind and focus on one single image. This could be a shape, a color, your favorite place or anything you associate with quiet and peace. It takes practice to avoid letting your mind wander to other things. Combine this technique with slow, deep breathing.

Progressive Relaxation - Lie in a comfortable position (on your back or on your side with bent knees are best). Close your eyes. Start by taking several deep, slow breaths. Now, as you breath in you are going to tense a muscle or muscle group, as you exhale let the muscle relax.
Follow this sequence:

> Inhale, flex your right foot.
> Exhale, let it relax.
> Inhale, flex your left foot.
> Exhale, let it go.

Repeat with the following contractions, inhaling and exhaling each time.

> Tighten both legs and press them together.
> Tighten the thighs.
> Tighten the buttocks.
> Pull in the abdominal area and flatten the back.
> Tense your chest and shrug the shoulders.
> Clench your fists and press your arms into the floor.
> Close your eyes tight and contract your facial muscles.

If you still feel tension in an area continue contracting and relaxing until the tightness disappears. Progressive relaxation trains your muscles to release tension as it builds up instead of storing it throughout the day.

Breathing - A simple deep breath or two can do wonders. Take time out for ten seconds when things get tense.

Be Good to Yourself - You only get one body and one life. Treat them right. You may need to make yourself an appointment in your calender for time to exercise or for something else that gives you pleasure. Other tactics include seeking help with time management, delegating responsibility and learning to say no. Remember that you are special. Focus on relaxation, enjoyment and health.

THE TOTAL WORKOUT

You now have the necessary information to design a safe and effective exercise program. Below is a summary of the components of a total workout (approximately 1 hour). If your time is limited, you can always warm-up, perform 20 minutes of aerobic activity, cool down and stretch. Muscle work can be done on alternate days. This fitness routine will fit easily into your lunch or other free time. On extremely busy days remember that something is better than nothing, a 15 minute walk will be beneficial even if it doesn't meet all of the criteria for true aerobic exercise.

Circulatory Warm-up (4 to 6 minutes)
Purpose: To increase core temperature and blood flow to the working muscles. Perform general activities at a low intensity level until you are perspiring lightly.

Stretching Warm-up (3 to 5 minutes)
Purpose: Mild static stretching to prevent injury.

Aerobic Activity (20 to 30 minutes)
Purpose: To maintain a heart rate within your individual target heart zone for a total of 20-30 minutes of continuous exercise. A bell curve pattern is recommended . Take part in aerobic activity at least 3 times per week.

Cool Down (3 to 10 minutes)
Purpose: Perform low-intensity, general movements until the heart rate falls below 120 beats per minute. Keep the feet and legs moving so that the blood will be pumped back toward the heart.

Muscular Strength and Endurance (10 to 20 minutes)
Purpose: Sufficient work on each muscle or muscle group to create overload. Concentrate on strengthening the weaker muscles. This segment can come before or after the aerobic activity. Calisthenics, stretchy bands, or weights can all be effective. Serious muscular training will take longer than 20 minutes.

Stretching and Relaxation (5 to 10 minutes)
Purpose: Static stretching for each muscle group designed to maintain or increase flexibility and relaxation exercises to release stress, anxiety and muscular tension.

THE FIVE MINUTE STRETCH

Follow this sequence for a safe, efficient flexibility workout. Remember to warm-up before you start, hold each position for at least 10 seconds and do not bounce. Close your eyes, take a few deep breaths and clear your mind. This is your time to relax.

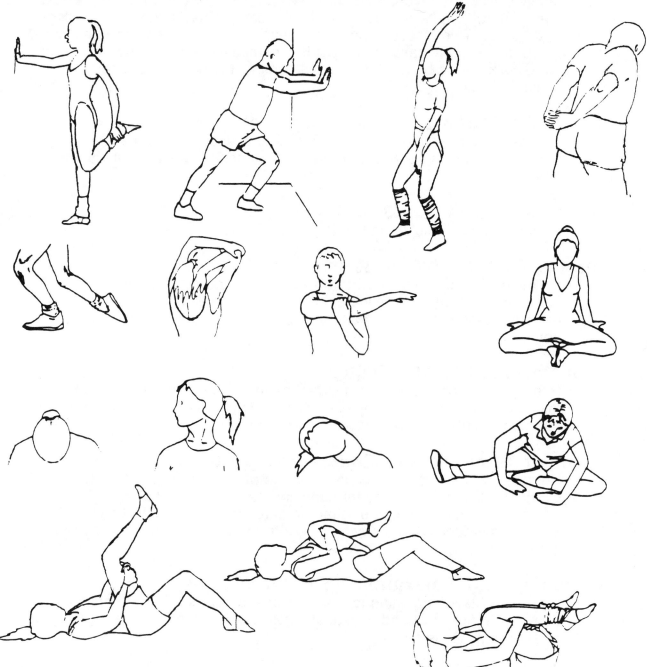

HEALTH & FITNESS ASSESSMENT

Name _____   **Age** _____yrs   **Sex**   M/F

Height _____'_____"   **Weight** _____lbs   **Goal** _____lbs

Blood Pressure _____systolic/_____diastolic   **Total Cholesterol** _____mg/dl

Circumferences Chest/Bust _____" Waist _____"   Hips _____" Thigh _____"

Three site skinfolds   (1)_____   (2)_____   (3)_____   Total_____

Body Fat Percentage _____%   **Body Fat Goal**_____%

Flexibility (sit and reach)   _____inches

Abdominal Strength (bent knee sit-ups in 1 minute)   _____sit-ups/minute

Upper Body Strength   (Push-ups in 30 seconds)   _____push-ups/30 seconds
             Circle one: regular or modified

Cardiovascular Endurance (Rockport walking test,   _____time
Cooper 1.5 mile walk/run, Cooper 12 minute walk/run,
3 minute step test, treadmill or bicycle test)   _____heart rate

The Karvonen Formula

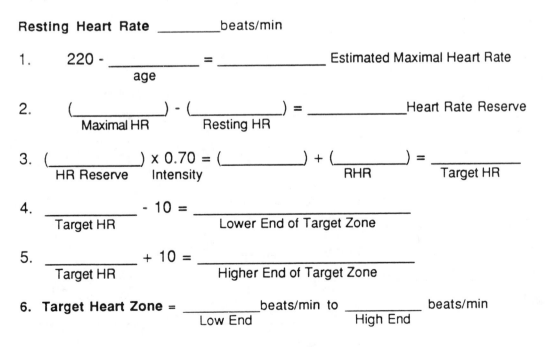

Resting Heart Rate _____beats/min

1.   220 - _____ = _____ Estimated Maximal Heart Rate
            age

2.   (_____) - (_____) = _____Heart Rate Reserve
        Maximal HR   Resting HR

3. (_____) x 0.70 = (_____) + (_____) = _____
      HR Reserve   Intensity   RHR   Target HR

4. _____ - 10 = _____
      Target HR   Lower End of Target Zone

5. _____ + 10 = _____
      Target HR   Higher End of Target Zone

6. **Target Heart Zone** = _____beats/min to _____ beats/min
                          Low End   High End

Personal Wellness Plan

Name _____ Date _____

Age _____ Sex _____ Height _____ ' _____ " Weight _____ lbs

General Wellness Goals _____

_____

_____

_____

Exercise Plan

Fitness Goals _____

_____

_____

Cardiovascular Fitness (see Chapter Four)

Activity: Circle activities that you like and that will fit into your lifestyle.

Walking	Road Cycling	Swimming	Low-impact Aerobics
Jogging	Stationary	Aqua-aerobics	High-impact Aerobics
	Cross Country Skiing		Other

Frequency _____ days/week

Duration _____ minutes within my Target Heart Zone

Intensity _____ % of Maximal Heart Rate Reserve

   Target Heart Zone _____ beats/min to _____ beats/min

   In 6 seconds   _____ to _____

   In 10 seconds _____ to _____

Muscular Strength and Endurance _____ days/week

Mode of exercise: calisthenics   light weights
                   stretchy bands   heavy weights

Include the following muscles and muscle groups:_____

_____

_____

_____

Perform _____ sets of_____ repetitions.
Choose a resistance such that you feel fatigue on the last 3–4 repetitions.

Flexibility _____ days/week

Perform slow, static stretching.
Hold each position 10–30 seconds.
Warm-up prior to stretching.

_____

_____

_____

Nutrition Plan

Nutrition Goals _____

_____

_____

My ideal weight is _____ lbs.

Stress Plan

Stress Management Goals _____

_____

_____

TOTAL WORKOUT LOG

	Example											
Date	5/2/89											
Circulatory Warm-up & Stretch	✓											
Type of Aerobic Activity *	W											
Minutes of Aerobic Activity	20											
Abdominals	2/15											
Upper Back	2/8/B											
Chest	2/10/60											
Hamstrings	2/10/30											
Biceps	2/10/B											
Triceps	2/10/B											
Deltoids	2/10/B											
Final Stretch and Relaxation	✓											

Muscle Strength and Endurance * *

Aerobic Activity In THZ

* W = Walk   S = Swim
   J = Jog   A = Aerobic Dance
   C = Cycle   O = Other

* * Sets/Repetitions/Resistance
(e.g., 2/10/25 = 2 sets of 10 repetitions with 25 pounds)
(e.g., 2/10/B = 2 sets of 10 repetitions with a stretchy band).